Taking the Work Out of Working Out

A Revolutionary Approach for Making Exercise More Exciting and Easier to Stick To

Charles Roy Schroeder, Ph.D.

Taking the Work Out of Working Out

Library of Congress Cataloging-in-Publication Data

Schroeder, Charles Roy
Taking the work out of working out / Charles Roy Schroeder.
p. cm.
Includes bibliographic references (p. 189) and index.
ISBN 1-56561-021-0 : $9.95
1. Exercise. 2. Senses and sensations. 3. Esthetics.
I. Title.
GV481.S29 1994
93-14776 613.7'1—dc20
CIP

Editor: Jeff Braun
Production Coordinator: Claire Lewis
Printed in the United States

10 9 8 7 6 5 4 3 2 1

Published by: CHRONIMED Publishing
P.O. Box 47945
Minneapolis, MN 55447-9727

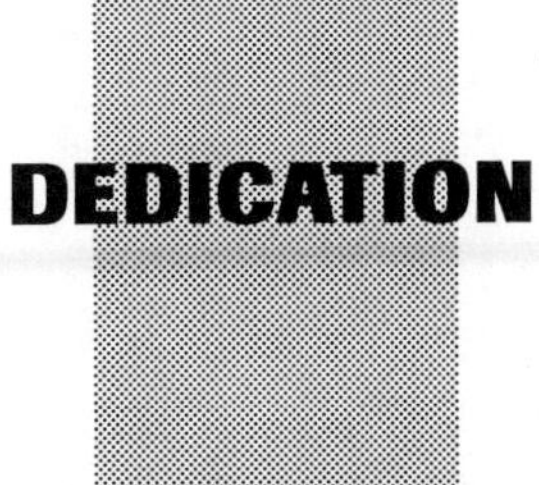

DEDICATION

To Anyone
Who Has Ever Disliked Exercise

ACKNOWLEDGMENTS

When in a rare egotistical frame of mind, I like to think the innovative approach to exercise presented in *Taking the Work Out of Working Out* is my idea and mine alone. In fact, in any frame of mind I would like to think that's true. The truth is, I owe a great deal to those who came before me in many academic areas—especially in philosophy, physiology, psychology, biomechanics, dance, and esthetics. These subjects provide the foundation for *Taking the Work Out of Working Out.*

One special person also deserves to be recognized for his contribution. David Williams, former chairman of the Music Department at Memphis State University, read the manuscript during its early stages and made many insightful suggestions. His encouragement—and friendship—is even more appreciated.

Any man who has been married for 30 years to a wonderful woman knows how valuable her loving support can be. My Judy's emotional support, alone, was extremely important. Of more practical importance, though, was her help on such countless mundane and frustrating matters such as proofreading and writing for photo, cartoon, and quotation permissions. When I say my wife is my right arm, it is only a slight exaggeration.

Editors are not always the most beloved and appreciated people in the eyes of authors. After all, they have the audacity to tinker with the "perfect" manuscripts offered by authors. Jeff Braun and Donna Hoel, my editors at CHRONIMED Publishing, were no exceptions. It really hurt my pride, though, when their gentle suggestions resulted in an improved manuscript. That humble admission on my part is reluctantly given. Of course, I'm kidding. I was delighted to have their ideas. They actually improved the manuscript a bit.

I reserve my greatest appreciation for the "big shots" at CHRONIMED Publishing. That, of course, would be the people who help select manuscripts for publication. I am thinking specifically of David "Der Wunderkind" Wexler, associate publisher, and Jon Ebersole, publisher. I knew, even before I typed the first word of *Taking the Work Out of Working Out,* that it would take a company with foresight, intelligence, and courage to publish this new approach to exercise. I am immensely grateful to CHRONIMED for being such a company.

ILLUSTRATIONS

* Line drawings by Rouse and Associates.

CONTENTS

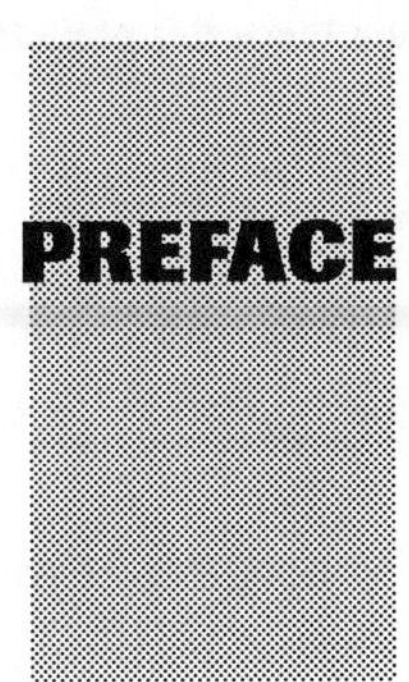

PREFACE

What is the most effective and natural way to take the work out of working out? Simple, BODY MUSIC! We all have it. Whenever you move, sensations arise from your muscles and joints. These internal feelings may be thought of as the body's music.

Like music, these feelings may or may not be pleasant. If they are randomly scattered sensations, the experience will be similar to listening to an orchestra tuning-up its instruments. Such chaotic sensory experiences, whether based on sound or exercise, will surely "get old fast."

On the other hand, if you know how to organize your movements into appealing patterns, the resulting sensations will be similar to the music of a finely conducted orchestra.

This book will help you choose movements that will convert your workouts into enjoyable, creative, sensual experiences—ones you will enthusiastically look forward to.

This innovative approach to exercise involves applying the principles of esthetics (creating and appreciating beauty) to physical activity. The methods are identical to those for all the arts from painting and music to cooking. The only difference is that exercise based on body music uses internal (kinesthetic) sensations instead of vision, sound, or taste.

With the body music method you do not merely work out, you create exciting, artistic events for your enjoyment. And because art is generally accepted as the ultimate activity of humanity, the artistic approach to exercise may be considered the ultimate concept of exercise.

This approach can be used by anyone involved in physical activity from novices to professional athletes, from aerobic dancers to bodybuilders to manual laborers. Body music can be integrated easily and comfortably with all exercise programs regardless of your goal, whether it is improved health, physical fitness, or appearance.

Because of the innovative nature of body music, an appropriate body of knowledge first has to be offered. In Part One, the three traditional reasons for exercising are explained and this new approach to exercise is introduced. Simple exercises are offered so you can begin to feel the sensations in the muscles and joints and organize them into pleasing artistic patterns. In Part Two, principles of physiology, psychology, and esthetics are presented to support the body music concept. Part Three gives many examples of how you can apply these methods to a variety of activities such as calisthenics, weight training, jogging, sports, and dance—and thereby create satisfying body music. Best of all, you are shown how to take the work out of working out.

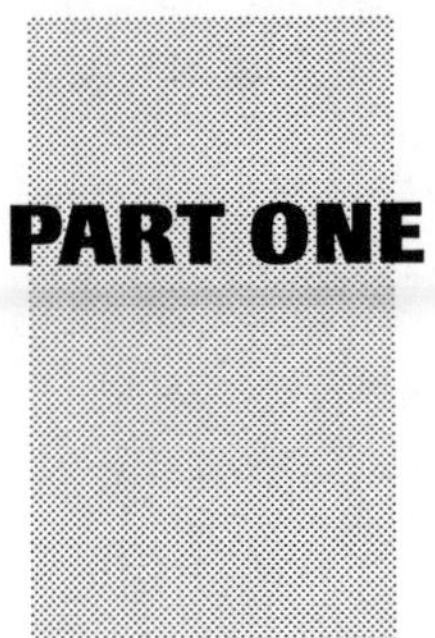

PART ONE

"It is art that makes life, makes interest, makes importance."
Henry James

DIMENSIONS OF EXERCISE

1

The three traditional approaches to exercise have been around for a long time. Specifically, physical activity has been used as (1) a kind of medicine, (2) as play, or (3) as an enjoyable sensory experience. There's nothing wrong with any of the three. But this book presents a far more effective and desirable concept of exercise for the first time, ever. Based on the internal sensations felt during exercise, this new concept does not interfere with any of the traditional approaches. In fact, it enhances them.

Exercise as Medicine

It's doubtful that primitive people engaged in formal exercise programs. They got plenty of physical activity just trying to survive by hunting and gathering and outrunning ugly, hostile neighbors. As civilizations became more complex and efficient, people had more leisure time and in general did not have to work as hard. This relaxed pace pleased them.

But lo! The more inactive individuals undoubtedly began to notice their bodies were not as strong as those of their harder working brothers and sisters, nor was their health as vital. And, to add insult to injury, their physiques were not as pleasing to the eye. To improve the situation wise men, called medicine men, may have suggested exercise programs for their sedentary members.

The prescribed exercises were probably unpleasant, and caused the clanspeople to cry, "Ugh, this is hard work!" They sweated. They groaned. They complained and probably even cursed. However, their health, fitness, and appearance did improve. At least it would have for those who were motivated or self-disciplined enough to stick with the programs.

But alas! As soon as people stopped exercising, their health, fitness, and appearance started to deteriorate. If they were perceptive, they would have exclaimed, "By Zorb! I'll have to do this all my life!" Of course, it was the rare individual who continued exercising throughout his or her entire life (an average of 26 years).

Exercise was a kind of medicine. Indeed, it was extremely good medicine, physiologically and psychologically, in both its preventive and therapeutic aspects. For most people, though, it was a foul tasting tonic. To make matters worse, a patient had to partake of it several times a week, and each draft lasted 30 to 60 minutes. It is no wonder that most of the people eventually stopped exercising.

Today, thousands of years later, we as a rule have more leisure time than ever. In addition, our jobs are less strenuous. As a result, relatively large numbers of men and women are engaging in exercise programs. Their reasons have not changed from those of primitive ancestors. We still want to increase our physical fitness, improve our health, and enhance our appearances. Modern wise men and women, called doctors, are prescribing exercise. It's still medicine.

In *American Health* (March, 1985), a report stated that almost 90 percent of all Americans who did any kind of exercise did so to improve their health, for weight control, to feel good, and to improve their fitness. Ninety percent! Things have not changed much in those thousands of years.

Exercise as medicine doesn't seem all that bad. But as mentioned before, it's difficult to persist for a lifetime at something perceived as medicine. How would *you* like to drink medicine for 30 or 60 minutes—three or four times a week—for your entire life?

Oh yes, people do exercise and they work hard at it. They sweat. They groan. They complain, and some even exclaim, "By God, I'll have to continue this all my life!" But they rarely do. It's no wonder Mark Twain said, "Exercise is loathsome."

People have long believed that something must be unpleasant to be good for them. This is the rationale behind the "no pain, no gain" philosophy currently spouted by exercise gurus. It's no wonder so many people don't exercise. Even the term we use for exercising is a turn-off. We are urged, for example, to "work out" by the health profession. Work out! The dreaded 'W' word.

In no other activity is the 'W' word used in reference to physical involvement. Most athletes, such as baseball players, *practice* to improve their skills. Dancers work as hard as other athletes—usually harder—but dancers never think of their exhausting sessions as working out. No, they *rehearse*. Gardeners *putter*. Piano players labor at a keyboard for hours but they don't call it working out—they *play* the piano. Well, I've tried to learn to play the piano. If that's play, 10 kilometer runs and grueling bodybuilding sessions are strolls through paradise.

Please allow me to digress for a moment to disclose a little known bit of history you'll no doubt find immensely fascinating. It has to do with the origin of the term "workout." One lovely Saturday morning in the not too distant past, a man told his wife he was going to *play* golf with his friends.

Now, the wife was a bit of a puritan and the word "play" to her was akin to fingernails screeching on a chalkboard. Her response was something like, "You what? If you want to play with something, Buster, you can play with this mop!" Poor fellow. He spent the day assisting his spouse with the housework. Mind you, I'm not suggesting that he should not have done otherwise.

The man's muscles ached while he mopped, vacuumed, and cleaned windows, but his keen mind was also hard at work. Seven days later he headed for the front door with his golf bag on his shoulder and a devious plan on his tongue. His mate (with arms imperiously folded across her chest) once again inquired as to his destination. He answered with a look of one whose soul is untarnished. "I'm going to work out, my little p-p-petunia."

"Work out?"

"Yeah, I'll be carrying this bag full of heavy clubs for about four or five miles up and down a bunch of steep hills all morning."

That sounded like a lot of work to her—and, in truth, it wouldn't be all that easy. "Okay, dear, when will you be home?" she asked with a satisfied smile.

This gentleman's cronies also had been experiencing marital discord because they were "playing" on Saturday mornings. As might be expected, the motley group also took to telling their wives that they were working out. To make a long story short, the term caught on—and continued to be used by men and women.

It would be nice if the historical account ended there. But the scheme backfired in the long run. Participants in many kinds of physical activity actually started to believe they were working—that they were exercising just to be healthier or to look better. They started to believe exercise was just a form of medicine they had to endure to achieve its benefits. All that attitude succeeded in doing, of course, was to take a lot of the fun out of the activities.

It's awful for anyone to think of exercise as medicine. Even worse, though, is to think of it as punishment. We've all seen physical education instructors and coaches who make their charges do push-ups or laps because of some rule infraction. Apparently those leaders think exercise is a medicine to cure rowdiness.

Not all physical educators and coaches use this technique to control students. My high school physical education teacher would punish misbehaving students by making them sit during the entire class period. I hated that; nearly everyone did. As a result, exercise was not viewed as punishment by us; it was considered a privilege. Unfortunately, that attitude is rare among today's students—and adults. Many people still think exercise is merely a type of medicine or punishment.

Exercise as Play

The maximum benefits of exercise, psychological as well as physiological, are achieved through lifelong participation. And to maintain this commitment, the proper attitude is necessary. Namely, exercise must not be viewed as an unpalatable medicine but as a fun experience. Exercise by nature is not loathsome, but the way in which it is approached can make it seem so.

Ideally, you should approach exercise sessions not with reluctance but with eager anticipation. There is no reason why you should not be able to. Indeed, it's natural to enjoy physical activity: Just watch young children gleefully at play (with minimal adult supervision).

Play, however, must not be thought of as being for children alone. Play is usually defined as something people do to amuse themselves. In no definition of play is age ever mentioned—and for good reason. People of all ages should play. The popular quotation which follows, by James Howell in *Proverbs,* is as true today as when it was set on paper in 1659. And it applies to everyone.

All work and no play makes Jack a dull boy.

Most adults take life too seriously. Playing forces us to focus on a pleasant activity. Forgotten is the distressing situation at work, the argument with a loved one, or the anxiety of an anemic bank account. It might be simpler just to say that play refers to anything that is fun to do. Clearly, the perception of exercise as play is a vast improvement over the perception of exercise as being just a form of medicine. Unfortunately, the *American Health* survey found that only 10 percent of the respondents exercised because they enjoyed it. Ten percent!

Ironically, the person who exercises because it's fun gets the most health benefits. When exercise is viewed as drudgery, neurochemicals associated with that attitude are secreted which block some of the health benefits.

Psychologist Ann McGee-Cooper, in her book, *You Don't Have to Go Home from Work Exhausted,* made an interesting point. Namely, your subconscious doesn't know the difference between real or imagined fun. Therefore, looking forward to the fun can give you the same energy boost as actually having fun. Conversely, viewing an upcoming exercise session as drudgery begins to drain you even before you start exercising.

It should be no great surprise that synonyms for drudgery include "toil," "work," "tedious *or* stupid *or* idiot *or* tiresome work," and "slavery." Sounds suspiciously close to "working out" doesn't it? Telling yourself all day that you are going to work out is not a great way to prepare yourself for the session. On the other hand, telling yourself you are going to play after work will probably put you in a very receptive mood for exertion.

It's important to remember:

We don't stop having fun when we're old;
We're old when we stop having fun.

Some people believe play is a lot more than just fun. I especially like John Huizinger's suggestion:

Play is one of the main bases of civilization.

Maybe so. Probably so! At any rate, the fun aspect of exercise must not be ignored.

While spontaneous activities such as skipping and playing tag may suffice as play for children, play for adults usually is more complex and formal. Sports are the most common examples. True, it's sometimes difficult to tell that players are enjoying themselves. The anger and expletives coming from upset participants are unmistakable signs of displeasure—the opposite of fun. That's kind of paradoxical, isn't it? They are supposed to be playing, but all they are feeling are hostility and anger. Out of curiosity I occasionally ask enraged players (enraged players of small stature, to be precise) if they are having fun. They don't seem to like the question, but it makes them think—I think.

Fortunately, sports and athletic games usually do make exercising more palatable by forcing participants to concentrate on competition, scoring points, and winning. All of these, like it or not, have come to be virtually synonymous with fun. Plus, there are the pleasant social aspects of sports and athletic games. Because most people consider exercise to be distasteful medicine, play does, indeed, help the "medicine go down."

Exercise as a Sensory Experience

Although play is a much more desirable goal of exercise than the dreaded 'W' word, there is a higher dimension. It's time to introduce the joyful 'K' word—kinesthesia. Just as people can be delighted by sensations of sight, sound, smell, and taste, they can also be delighted by kinesthesia.

Kinesthesia is the internal sensation created when the body moves. It's the basis of *body music*. Kinesthesia is often called the "muscle sense," but that's misleading because kinesthesia arises from joints and tendons as well as from muscles. When a muscle contracts or when movement occurs, receptors are stimulated and nerve impulses are sent to the brain.

The brain interprets the incoming signals and determines how the movement feels. These feelings are called kinesthetic sensations, which is just a variation of the 'K' word. Slide your lower jaw from side to side; the sensations you feel will be kinesthetic sensations. If you change the speed or the direction of sliding, the sensations will vary.

There are countless other examples. You'll be able to think of many yourself, but a few are mentioned here to help you become aware of your kinesthesia. Because you're probably sitting as you read this book, extend your legs. Vary the degree of extension, the speed of movement, and the resistance if you have some ankle weights available. By concentrating on the kinesthesia you'll detect widely varying sensations. You can also press your palms together in front of your chest, lean from side to side at the waist, press your upper arms against your sides, suck-in your abdomen, or extend your arms to the sides and do arm circles.

Another example of kinesthesia that is as delightful as it is commonplace and natural is a yawn. Just reading about the act may inspire you to "cut loose." If so, go right ahead but make sure you *concentrate* on the yawn. As some muscles contract and others stretch, including those around your eyes and mouth, concentrate on the internal sensations—your body music.

Even if everyone felt the same or similar kinesthesia for each exercise, exactly how a particular movement is *perceived* varies considerably. The kinesthesia of walking up stairs, for instance, may be viewed with displeasure by one person. Another may find the sensations exceedingly pleasant. While the sensory input to the brain may be identical for both individuals, the evaluations will be colored by previous learning experiences. Because no two people have identical learning experiences, the kinesthetic feelings will be perceived in different ways.

Infants and young children revel in the kinesthesia of physical activity. As they grow older they are taught by their elders that exercise is good for them, which, ironically, may lead to negative feelings and attitudes toward exercise. Everyone knows, seemingly instinctively, that if something is good for you it cannot possibly taste, sound, or feel good. By adulthood these negative feelings are usually firmly entrenched and difficult to change.

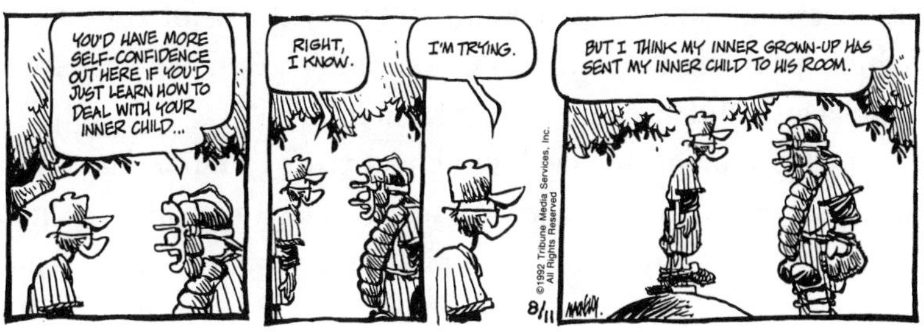

SHOE reprinted by permission: Tribune Media Services.

Fortunately, only the thought of exercise is distasteful to people—not the kinesthesia itself. Actually, nearly every adult has forgotten that the sense even exists—its pleasure having been long veneered with the attitude that exercise is medicinal.

If people don't enjoy their kinesthesia, they're not likely to exercise very much. How long would you listen to music if it were ear-splitting and discordant (assuming you're not a teenager)? How long would you munch on bitter strawberries? How long would you wear woolen underwear? More to the point, how long would you exercise if the associated kinesthesia was unpleasant? The answers to all the above questions are obvious: "not for long." The secret to keeping people involved in physical activity is simple—help them enjoy their body music and maximize that enjoyment.

Because most adults don't even know they have a kinesthetic sense, they don't have feelings toward it one way or the other. How could they? Because of this unawareness, the task of helping them to once again enjoy their kinesthesia may not be all that difficult. Convincing people they actually have kinesthesia is the first step.

That may strike you as being rather strange. Logically, you would think we would be aware of all our sensations. But we are not. Part of the problem is that the other senses are usually much stronger and capture our attention at the expense of kinesthesia, which generally has more subtle sensations. Besides, a sensation can be quite intense and still be ignored.

Quite often during my high school years I would play basketball with friends after school. We weren't allowed to play in shoes, (those were the days before the ubiquitous sneakers), so we'd play in our socks. After about 30 minutes we'd stop for water. Only when the concentration of play was broken did we realize we had very large, painful blisters on our feet. Watching a herd of skinny, half-naked boys racing toward a water fountain while running on their heels and elbowing each other is a sight no one should miss.

Kinesthetic sensations, too, can be very intense and a person can still be unaware of them. As an illustration, watch a person straining to complete a set of heavy arm curls. Intense and powerful kinesthetic sensations are being evoked. But when you ask him how the kinesthesia felt, he probably won't know what you're talking about. Most people have to be educated to experience kinesthesia. This can be done through an effective program of movement experiences.

The next step is probably most difficult. It's to help people develop positive perceptions of the body music associated with exercise. These perceptions can be learned. The ease of learning depends on many factors including your 1) *initial* kinesthetic perceptions, which can range from negative to neutral to positive, 2) *confidence* in the kinesthetic approach to exercise, and 3) *philosophical* framework. A hedonist, for example, will have little difficulty in relating to and accepting this kinesthetic approach. A puritan, on the other hand, is likely to feel uncomfortable with any pleasurable feelings.

In their book, *Healthy Pleasures,* Robert Ornstein and David Sobel said humans evolved to seek pleasure to assure survival. That, no doubt, applies to *all* animals. What better way, they asked, is there to motivate vital survival functions, such as eating and sexual reproduction, than by making the activities enjoyable? The authors say most of us are not getting our daily requirement of sensual pleasures. They also suggest that modern life has deprived us of too many of these delights—and balance needs to be regained.

Ornstein and Sobel wrote about the importance of pleasures through sight, sound, touch, taste, and hearing sensations—but they overlooked kinesthesia. They can be forgiven, however, because nearly everyone does overlook it. This book does not! It shows you how to increase your enjoyment of exercise by focusing on your body music, making your exercise sessions feel good, and therefore making your life happier.

Exercise as Art

The concept of exercise introduced in this book, however, is not limited merely to helping you enjoy your kinesthesia. A giant leap beyond that level is achieved by showing how you can consciously arrange your kinesthetic sensations into artistic patterns—based on the law of esthetics.

As explained earlier, kinesthetic receptor organs send impulses to the brain, which interprets them as sensations. You can create kinesthetic art by organizing the sensations into esthetically pleasing patterns. All you have to do is simply control your movements, just as a painter controls the application of colors to a canvas. Exercise approached in this way becomes an artistic, kinesthetic event.

Such exercise becomes art because it meets the three criteria of art. That is, the kinesthesia of exercise 1) can be *perceived* through the senses, 2) can be organized toward a *unified experience,* and 3) can result in an *esthetic* event. This approach to exercise requires some cerebral activity, but that's okay; the best exercise is that which employs the mind pleasantly.

There are many definitions of art. Donald Kuspit, in his 1993 book, *The Cult of the Avant-Garde*, said, "True art makes people feel inwardly alive." Kurt Vonnegut felt that everyone should be an artist. He said a person didn't have to be good as long as he or she got pleasure. What a great idea! Using Vonnegut's definition, everyone can be a kinesthetic artist. They don't have to be good as long as they get pleasure. As a result, in creating an artistic experience you no longer merely work out. You create body music and thereby become a kinesthetic artist—or more succinctly, a kinoartist (another variation of the 'K' word).

I have helped many people become kinoartists in the university physical activity classes I have taught over the years, ranging from weight training and dance to boxing and juggling. Students not only enjoy the activities far more as kinoartists, but they improve their fitness and skills faster because the activities are fun.

No, kinoartists do not merely work out. They practice to improve their abilities to produce an esthetic event. Because art is the ultimate exercise of humanity, kinoart is the ultimate approach to exercise. Ultimate, of course, means "the very best." This lofty objective, however, does *not* mean kinoartists cannot get the traditional physical benefits of exercise. On the contrary, kinoartists should be more successful in obtaining them. But they'll have vastly more rewarding and uplifting exercise experiences. The chief aim of this book, simply, is to show you how to become a kinoartist.

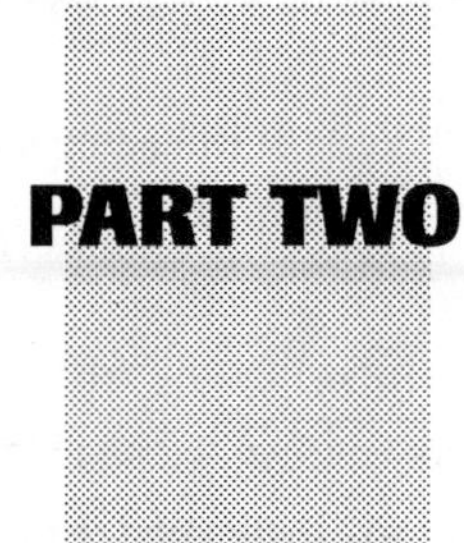

PART TWO

"Art necessarily presupposes knowledge"
John Stuart Mill

For every artist, including a kinoartist, a specific body of knowledge is required as a springboard to creativity. Michelangelo suggested this beautifully in one of his sonnets on the act of creativity.

When that which is divine in us doth try
To shape a face, both brain and hand unite. . .

Rodin expressed the thought more simply by saying,

Not for a moment can an artist get along without science.

Information does not necessarily have to be obtained through teachers and books. In truth, these formal methods sometime impede learning. When used effectively, however, they do tend to be more complete, more organized, and more efficient in conveying information.

No matter how it is acquired, artists must have some knowledge of their medium—and the more they know the better. Painters, for instance, must know such basics as the best thinners and how to prepare various surfaces such as canvas, wood, and plaster. Knowing how to mix colors to achieve variations in hue, value, and intensity is also necessary. The list goes on and on, as it does for other artists including choreographers, musical composers, sculptors, architects, and chefs.

Incidentally, all of these artists are in an enviable position because everyone accepts their works as art. First of all, people can *see* paintings, sculpture, architecture, and dance. They can *hear* music and *taste* culinary creations. Secondly, people have been taught all their lives that these sensory experiences are esthetically stimulating and can be thought of as art.

On the other hand, until now the public has never been taught that the kinesthetic sensations associated with exercise could ever have esthetic appeal. Understandably, the concept may seem far-fetched. After all, kinesthesia is a very personal internally directed sense, which is not nearly as obvious as the externally directed senses of sight, hearing, taste, smell, and touch.

Because the idea of kinoart is so new, there are no traditional foundations for this creative activity. One of the first orders of business, therefore, is to establish such foundations. We need to learn about our bodies and the music they can make. And that's the purpose of this Part Two.

KINESTHETIC SENSATIONS

2

Without our senses we could not survive. Without our senses there would be little reason to want to. At best they bring beauty, joy, and spice into our lives. At worst they bring pain and ugliness, but even then our senses at least let us know we are alive.

Unfortunately, many people feel half alive because they're not in touch with the myriad sensory experiences that swirl around and within them. Who would want to feel half alive? It also means half dead. Why don't people simply allow the sensations to flood their consciousness? Perhaps because some effort is often required. In other words:

You may have to bend over to smell the roses.

Such effort is certainly true for body music. Some people may be too apathetic to make the effort, but most are probably just not aware of the delightful varieties and subtleties of the sensations available to them. The problem, therefore, is essentially a lack of knowledge—and that can be solved simply by providing pertinent information.

The aim of this chapter is to help you understand and appreciate your kinesthetic senses. Here it is clearly established that kinesthesia does exist and that it is an important sense not only in its own right but in its alliance with the other senses. General principles of sensation are also discussed with the emphasis, naturally, being on kinesthesia. This familiarization is the foundation of knowledge you will need to become a kinoartist.

Sense Organs

The body's senses let you know what is happening within and around your body. The outposts of the senses are called receptors. These tiny organs respond to specific stimuli such as light, sound, heat, cold, pressure, smell, taste, pain, joint movements, and muscle tension.

Each sensory receptor is attached to the end of a nerve fiber, called a neuron. When a receptor is stimulated, an electrical impulse is generated in its neuron. The impulse travels along the neuron to the brain. Interestingly, the nature of every nerve impulse is exactly the same no matter what kind of stimulus produced it. That is, neurons from heat receptors do not carry heat to the brain, nor do neurons from the eyes carry light. The impulses are always electrical.

How, then, are you able to experience different sensations? It all depends on where a sensory impulse ends in your brain. For example, the optic nerve leads from the eyes to the rear of the brain's outer layer (cortex). Electrical impulses to this area are interpreted as vision. The sensations of kinesthesia and touch arise from impulses that go to the area of the brain's cortex that is located above the ears.

Fascinatingly, if your kinesthetic neurons ended in the optical portion of the brain, their impulses would also be interpreted as vision. One has to wonder what sights would be created by the kinesthesia of a basketball shot, a karate kick, or a gymnastics routine.

Kinesthesia

Our senses are commonly classified as sight, hearing, taste, and the somatic (body) senses. The latter category includes the sense of touch, warmth, cold, pain, and kinesthesia.

As stated previously, kinesthetic receptors are found in skeletal muscles, tendons, and especially joints. The body has more than 200 joints. Impulses from these receptors enable your brain to rapidly and accurately determine joint angles and the positions of body parts. Other receptors, which also give rise to kinesthesia (body music), allow the brain to determine tensions in muscles and tendons.

While the senses are usually discussed separately, far more important are the relationships between them. For instance, it has long been recognized that people "taste" more with their noses and even their eyes than their taste buds. This is why a cherry flavored drink that is colored green will usually be identified by a taster as lemon or lime. It also explains why most people would "pass" on mashed potatoes dyed purple.

Humans, except for the blind, are strongly sight oriented. Because vision is such an attention-grabbing sense, kinesthesia goes unnoticed by most people. However, it is constantly on the job. Eyes, for instance, get credit for judging distances, but this important skill actually depends on highly sensitive kinesthetic receptors in the six small muscles that move each eyeball.

As you look at this page, your eyes are not exactly parallel because the muscles cause each eye to angle inwardly to some degree. The angle varies with the distance of your eyes from the words. If the brain knows these angles from past experiences, it can estimate the distance to this page. Because the angles are not supplied directly to the brain, it has to determine the angles from the kinesthetic sensations it receives from the eye muscles. This calculation of distance is remarkable enough when an object is stationary. It's vastly more complicated, though, when a batter have to determine the rate of changing distances (speed) of a ball hurtling toward home plate—and to do it fast enough to hit the ball.

The inner ear is generally known to help us maintain balance. However, receptors in the eyes, pressure receptors on the bottom of the feet, and kinesthetic receptors throughout the body are also involved.

Even kinesthesia's cousin, the sense of touch, cheats kinesthesia of its share of credit. Most people think touch allows them to judge the weight of an object, as well as its firmness, size, and shape (especially when one's eyes are closed). Kinesthesia, as you may have guessed by now, actually has the primary role in all these functions. For example, when an object such as a peach is placed in your hand, its weight will cause some deformation of the skin. From pressure receptors in the skin, the brain can roughly estimate the fruit's firmness. But a far more accurate appraisal of the peach's firmness results when you gently squeeze it between your fingers and thumb. Tension in the muscles and tendons of the fingers increases. The degree of tension detected by kinesthetic receptors enables the brain, based upon past experiences, to determine the peach's firmness.

A similar process occurs when you hold an object to measure its weight, or run your hands over it to determine its size and shape. In estimating an object's weight, kinesthetic receptors sensitive to tension in the muscles and tendons are primarily involved.

In determining on object's size and shape, the main kinesthetic receptors are those sensitive to joint position and movement. As always, your brain compares the sensory input with previous experiences in making its evaluations. These kinesthetic sensations explain why sculpture is considered so sensuous. In fact, Eskimos create small sculptures that aren't meant to be seen; they are only meant to be caressed. Because kinesthesia is the basis of the sensuousness of sculpture, it's easy to understand how kinesthetic sensations have such great sensual potential.

Kinesthetic assistance in sensory experiences is not a one-way street. The other senses can enrich the feelings of body music. While bicycle riding, you typically feel a generalized joy of movement. If you concentrate on your leg muscles, you'll realize some of the sensation comes from the rhythmic changes of muscle tension. By shifting your attention to the knees and ankles as they alternately extend and flex, you will become aware of a different but still enjoyable feeling. In other words, both muscle and joint sensations contribute to the total body music you will be experiencing.

Next, divert your attention to the pressure of your feet against the pedals, or to the gentle vibrations in your body as the tires roll over the finely pebbled surface of the road. The cool wind flowing over your skin and tousling your hair adds a further satisfying touch as does the texture of clothes as they caress your skin. By pedaling fast enough, acidic wastes in the leg muscles increase and produce an exquisite burning sensation that adds a dash of spice to the body music.

In brief, kinesthetic sensations can be greatly enhanced by other sensory experiences. This fact should not be forgotten if you want to convert your exercise sessions into enjoyable esthetic events—and become a kinoartist.

A Receptive Body

Although all of the sense organs send information in the form of electrical impulses to the brain, a great many variations are possible because for most senses there are several kinds of receptors. For vision this results in different colors. Similarly, there are different sounds and different smells. Just think of the wide variety of tastes that are possible, and there are only four different kinds of receptors on your tongue (sweet, sour, bitter, and salty).

Body music is no different. There are several types of kinesthetic receptors and a unique feeling is associated with each. This variety, of course, gives you an infinitely rich keyboard to create your body music.

Furthermore, within each sensory system there are differences in sensitivity. Skin surfaces on different parts of the body, for instance, have different sensitivities to temperature, touch, and pain. The tongue, too, is divided into regions that are particularly sensitive to one taste or another.

By the same token, you may recognize your body's music more easily in some muscles and joints than in others. The quality of body music will likewise vary. This explains, in part, why a bodybuilder will enjoy one exercise over another, and one level of resistance over another for the same movement.

More than likely, the kinesthetic sensations you feel for a specific muscular tension and joint movement are very similar to those felt by another person. At least, such similarity is experienced in the other senses. Red is seen as red to most people; candy tastes sweet to most people; and F sharp sounds like F sharp to most people.

But there are differences among individuals. Some people have perfect pitch detection and others are tone deaf. While some people can identify colors very accurately, others are color blind. Undoubtedly, this applies to body music, too. A small percentage of people will be acutely aware of their body music, a like percentage will feel nothing, and the vast majority will fall somewhere between the two extremes.

Your ability to "hear" your body music may also be affected by stronger sensations that drown out, or mask, the kinesthesia. A common example is pain that is so intense that it completely overrides lesser pains. In like fashion, powerful contractions of one muscle group will tend to mask the kinesthesia of gently contracting muscles. As an aspiring kinoartist, you should avoid such masking. Richer body music will usually be created if the sensations from one muscle group are not allowed to completely mask those of others.

Loud sounds or bustling people can also cause masking. Beginning kinoartists are particularly susceptible to this type of overriding because they are unlikely to have a keen awareness of their body music to begin with. Therefore, you should practice in an environment uncluttered with distractions so you can concentrate more easily on your kinesthesia. If distractions cannot be avoided, it helps to close your eyes and use earplugs. You may get puzzled looks, but—who cares? Selected stimuli such as music can eventually be introduced into practice sessions to enhance the kinesthetic experience.

Practical Applications

Many practical applications can be made from the information in this chapter. For instance, you now realize you can create and control a dazzlingly large number of kinesthetic sensations. With practice that number can be increased in many ways. More specifically, body music can be varied:

1) by *contracting* different muscles or combinations of muscles
2) by *stretching* muscles
3) by moving different joints or *combinations* of joints
4) by varying the *speed* of movements
5) by varying the *resistance* against movements

You will probably find that moderate muscular contractions will create the most pleasant sensations. Weak efforts will produce barely discernible sensations while extreme exertions may cause unpleasant or even painful feelings, as in the case of muscle cramps. Only through trial and error can you determine the intensity of effort that feels most desirable from your kinesthetic viewpoint. As you become more experienced, you will come to appreciate the nuances of effort from very weak to very powerful contractions in a wide range of movements.

Because of individual differences, not everyone will attain the same kinesthetic success. As in any artistic medium, some will reach high artistic plateaus; others will not. Still, virtually everyone is capable of improving his or her kinoartistic abilities. Exercise sessions will cease to be drudging "work outs." Instead, they will become highly satisfying, creative experiences.

KINESTHETIC PERCEPTIONS

3

As already mentioned, specific sensations look, sound, or taste about the same for everyone. Why is it, then, that some children love furry puppies while others are terrified of them? The answer is perception.

The brain gives meaning to sensory information based on previous experiences. A child who loves puppies undoubtedly has had pleasant experiences with puppies. The fearful child, on the other hand, undoubtedly had negative experiences. Perhaps an overly anxious parent snatched the child away from an energetic puppy, or the animal barked loudly and scared the child. These are obvious examples, but all past experiences help to determine how a person perceives an event or sensation.

That's not to imply that we are prisoners of our perceptions. On the contrary, the perception of nearly every sensation can be changed. It's possible, for instance, to help a child who is frightened of dogs to love them. It's also possible to design experiences to increase the strength of kinesthetic perceptions and to improve one's feeling about them. These abilities are particularly important for aspiring kinoartists because they must be able to control their perceptions. Therefore, the first order of business is to learn how perception relates to kinoart.

Nature vs. Nurture

There are many theories of perception. For the most part, they are divided between nature and nurture. Naturists believe people perceive their environment (internal and external) based on their genetic make-up. An example is our innate perception of depth.

Nurturists, on the other hand, believe perceptions are learned, that people organize and interpret sensations strictly on the basis of previous experiences. How people perceive dogs is an example.

A wedding of the two theories is probably the most sensible position. Applied to kinoart, that means some kinesthetic sensations tend to be innately pleasant while others may be innately unpleasant. That would explain why bodybuilders tend to prefer the sensations associated with bench pressing much more than those associated with leg extensions or squats. How anyone perceives any of the kinesthetic sensations, though, can be greatly modified by personal experiences—including training. Many useful techniques are suggested in this and subsequent chapters.

With body music and other sensory experiences, the first exposure consists of little more than the ability to *detect* or become aware of a sensation. With repeated encounters, people gradually find they are able to *recognize* differences and similarities between sensations. Eventually they are able to *identify* sensations and *perceive* some meaning, or feeling, for them.

Only after many repetitions of a kinesthetic sensation will you typically be able to identify it as one you have felt before. This suggests that kinoartists, as do other artists, must practice diligently to develop their perceptual abilities. The more you practice the more accurately you will identify the sensations and expand your body music repertoire.

Eventually, you'll be able to promptly and reliably reproduce the sensations at will, just as violinists learn to coax specific notes from their instruments. Ultimately, your kinesthetic sensations will have meanings and emotions attached to them. When that occurs, you will be creating and enjoying artistic kinesthetic experiences while you are exercising—whether lifting weights, dancing, or raking leaves.

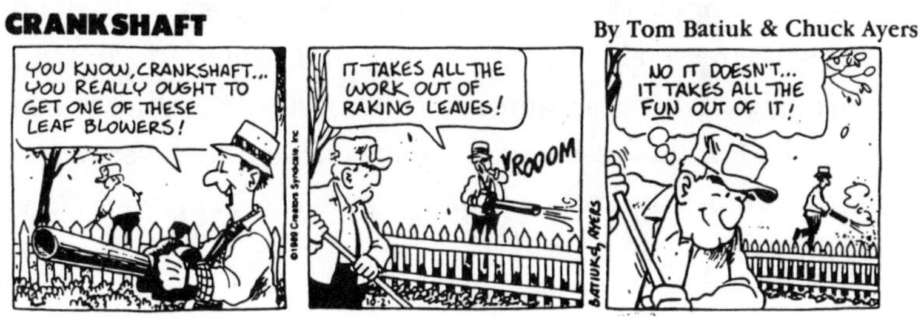

Virtually everyone who studies perceptions believes:

The whole is greater than the sum of its parts.

That is, sensations, typically, do not remain separate and distinct. When you listen to music, for example, the many notes (parts) taken by themselves do not mean very much; however, they blend to produce a completely new perceptual effect that *does* have meaning.

In the body music associated with a tennis serve, the "parts" refer to the individual kinesthetic sensations produced by each muscle and joint that moves. When a serve is properly performed, however, the player will not usually be aware of any individual sensations. Instead, he or she will experience a totally different perceptual effect as the separate sensations blend into a smooth, rhythmic sequence. This "whole" results in body music.

One of the most significant aspects of a stimulus, such as exercise, is its *ideal* complexity—a level of complexity most people prefer. People usually will not choose a stimulus that is simpler than the ideal—it is too boring. On the other hand, through design or chance, people will occasionally deal with a slightly more complex stimulus than the ideal. If the experience is satisfying, the more complex stimulus will then become the new ideal one. For example, skaters, gymnasts, and jugglers consistently attempt progressively difficult stunts, and skiers are drawn to increasingly challenging slopes. Ideal complexity applies to body music, too. For this reason you are encouraged to advance from simple to more complex kinesthetic experiences. This book shows you how.

Auditioning the Sensations

You are never aware of all of the sensations that arrive at your brain at any point of time. Thank goodness! There's just too much. Total awareness would leave you hopelessly confused. The brain wisely *selects* the sensations it wishes to pay attention to—according to your immediate needs and interests.

Even while reading this page, you may be completely unaware of some objects in the room and perhaps the conversation of nearby people or the tapping motion of your own foot. This ability of selective attention helps you concentrate more effectively on important tasks. Selective attention, conscious as well as unconscious, also helps you, as a kinoartist, eliminate irrelevant or conflicting sensations from kinesthetic creations.

People often err in the selection of stimuli. These errors explain why tricky maneuvers are so successful in athletics. For instance, basketball players will frequently fake a jump shot to get the defender off-balanced and then drive-in for a lay-up. The victim is simply tricked into selecting the wrong stimuli to respond to.

Kinoartists, too, must choose movements with care. One of their chief errors will be in concentrating on the kinesthetic sensations of only one or two muscle groups at a time. This limitation will reduce the richness and depth of their body music. Another error is to rush through a movement. The brain does not have enough time to fully grasp the kinesthetic nuances. This can be compared to connoisseurs gulping down vintage champagne, (which they would never do). Connoisseurs swish the wine gently around the mouth while they concentrate on its flavor, bouquet, and other sensual qualities. Kinoartists can learn a lot from connoisseurs and, in fact, from artists in every type of medium.

One of the most effective ways to capture a person's sensory attention is to create an abrupt change. In the previous reading situation, for instance, if the blocked-out conversation abruptly becomes much louder or much softer you would be jolted into an awareness of the sound.

More to the point are bicyclists who pedal along a level road at a steady, moderate pace. They may be oblivious to the body music of pedaling until the road rapidly begins to incline or decline. Moreover, the greater the change, the greater the probability that they will become aware of the kinesthesia. Kinoartists can use abrupt changes to create more satisfying body music.

People perceive according to their own interests. This is clearly demonstrated every time a football game runs over its scheduled time on television. Die-hard fans will not be concerned about how the overrun might affect subsequent programming and may even be unaware of the extended duration of the game. On the other hand, people who *are* interested in watching the program that follows the game will be acutely aware of the time extension and may flood the television station with protests. In the same vein, people who have an interest in kinoart are far more likely to be conscious of their kinesthetic sensations and its subtle variations than those who have little or no interest.

A popular adage states:

You only see what you want to see.

That is not entirely true, but the tendency does exist. As a matter of fact, when a person wants to see something more clearly, the brain automatically orders the pupils of the eyes to dilate to admit more light. For confirmation of this, show a man a picture of a voluptuous woman and closely watch his pupils. The term "eye opener" will immediately be observed. The picture of a nude man would undoubtedly have the same effect on most women. Why do you think *Cosmopolitan* occasionally resorts to male centerfolds? They are hoping that eye-opening will lead to purse-opening.

Not only for sight, but for all the senses, people perceive more clearly those things they *want* to perceive. In fact, they may perceive a particular sensation without even receiving a stimulus if the desire is strong enough.

Imagine a sailor at sea in a thick fog who wants to gain the safety of a harbor before a storm strikes. Assume that a bell buoy marks the entrance to the harbor. Because he wants so much to hear the bell, the sailor, typically, will "hear" it several times before he is actually within auditory range. People are also much more likely to perceive their body's music if they really want to. Furthermore, the greater the desire, the stronger the perception tends to be.

It appears that once people become attuned to their kinesthetic sensations, the need to experience them approaches addiction—a healthy addiction. It may be based on physiological or psychological factors or a combination of the two; no one knows for sure. In any case, a confirmed exerciser can be expected to crave movement and muscular exertion after he or she is sedentary for more than a few days.

Kinesthetic perceptions are also influenced by how the information is organized by the brain. People generally perceive objects as figures against a background. In observing a pastoral scene, for instance, a solitary tree in the foreground will appear as a figure and the remainder of the scene will be the ground. This figure-ground relationship occurs in all of the senses.

In swimming, the kinesthetic "figure" could be the sensations from the swimmer's powerfully contracting shoulder muscles. The "ground" would be the body music coming from the other joints and muscles. Even though the body music of "figure" movements is more noticeable, kinoartists should broaden their attention to include the more subtle "ground" body music, which can be very appealing. Incidentally, if you are a swimmer, try closing your eyes for several strokes at a time. You'll be amazed at the diversity of your kinesthesia and how clearly it is perceived. I guarantee it to be a fascinating sensory experience—and a surprisingly intense one.

Another factor, closure, refers to the tendency of a person to perceive an incomplete objective as a complete one. For the sense of vision this is illustrated with an incomplete drawing of the animal depicted in Fig. 3-1.

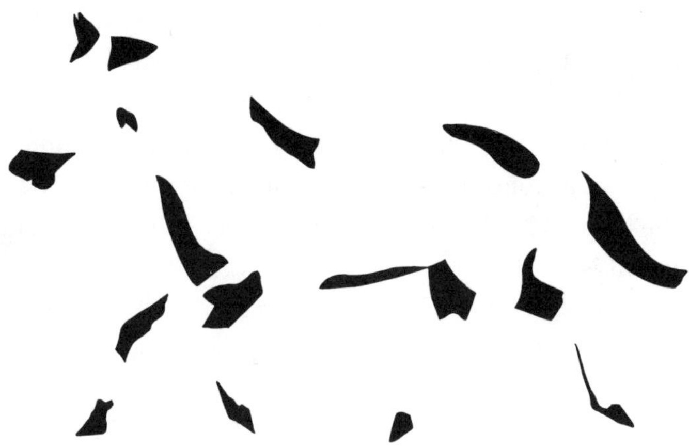

Fig. 3-1. A Visual Example of Closure.

For a kinesthetic example of closure, consider a boxer's demonstration of one of his bouts; he typically uses half blows similar to shadow boxing. Even though the punches are only partial, the boxer will falsely perceive them as being kinesthetically complete. This perceptual error of closure is not likely to occur in the actual fight, though. Visual cues, such as the distance between him and his opponent, serve to override and eliminate the phenomenon.

Other athletes are not so fortunate. In shotputting, for example, there are two distinct phases, the slide across the circle and the put itself. Any hesitation between the two phases shortens the distance of the put. Yet, the most common error in shotputting is this hesitation. This problem is difficult to correct because most shotputters are unaware of the pause. Because of closure, they perceive the two phases as being one complete movement and it is difficult to convince them otherwise.

Closure also has an adverse effect on a kinoartist's creative efforts. When abbreviated movements are perceived as being complete, the kinesthesia will be lacking some of the sensations of full movement. The sensory experience, therefore, will not be as full-bodied as it could be. For this reason, as a kinoartist, you should generally make your movements complete.

Another aspect of kinesthetic perception is the tendency for sensations that are in close proximity, in time or location, to be perceived as a group. This explains why the form in Fig. 3-2 looks like the letter "H" when in reality the upper half is a "W" and the lower half is an "M."

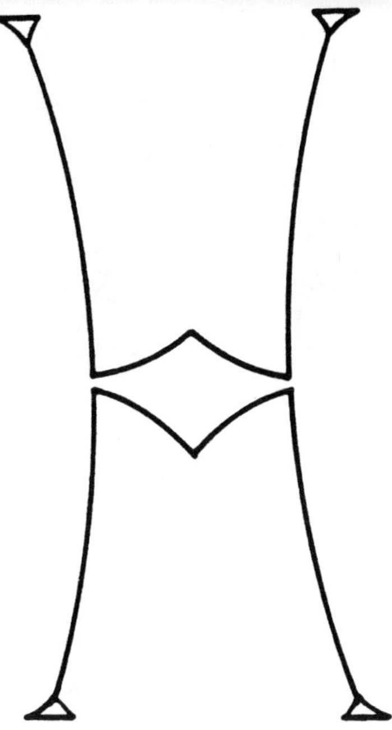

Fig. 3-2. A Visual Example of Proximity.

When a person jumps vertically (Fig. 3-3A) using only the muscles of his legs and arms, he will usually feel two distinct sensations because of the distance between the limbs. With practice the sensations may eventually be perceived as a unit. You can hasten the kinesthetic fusion by linking the arm and leg movements with properly synchronized movements of the back as shown in (B). This produces a unified sensation that will have more esthetic appeal than the two seemingly unrelated kinesthetic patterns produced by the arm and leg movements alone.

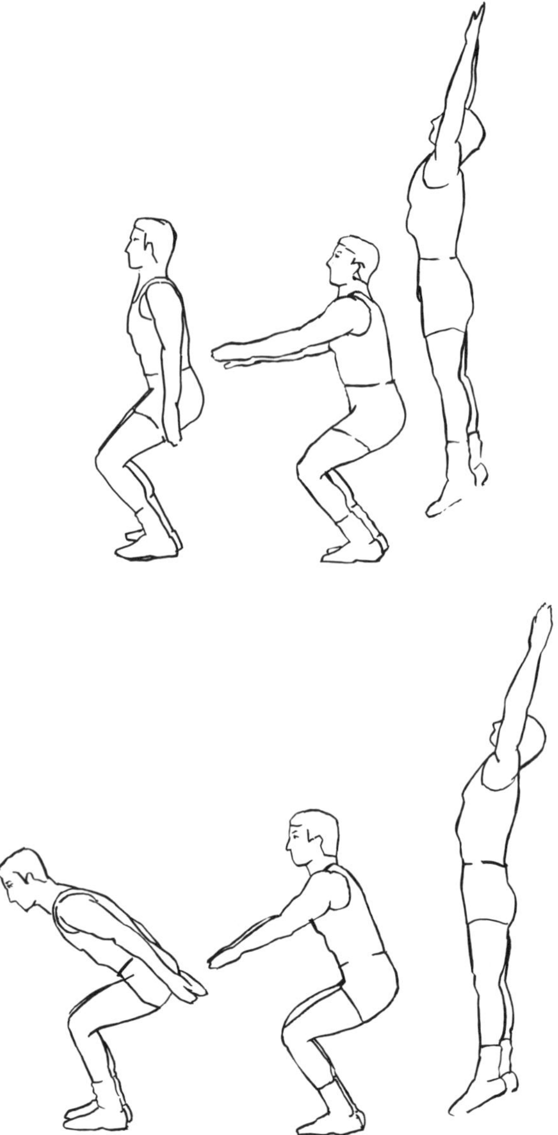

Fig. 3-3. A Kinesthetic Example of Proximity.

It is much easier for the brain to organize sensations into a single perceptual unit if their characteristics are similar. For example, when a person juggles three balls of identical size, shape, and weight, the activity will be experienced as a complex but single kinesthetic event.

On the other hand, when three different objects such as a large ring, a juggling club, and a ping pong ball are juggled, the activity may never be viewed as a single kinesthetic unit—no matter how much one practices. The objects are so dissimilar and each toss so different that the event will probably always be perceived as three distinct groups of kinesthetic sensations. Which of the two kinds of juggling is kinesthetically more enjoyable? It depends largely on the expertise of the juggler. A beginner will find the sensations associated with juggling dissimilar objects to be chaotic. The more proficient a person becomes, however, the more he or she will enjoy the more complex body music.

This discussion of organization is not meant to suggest any particular movement is superior to another. It is impossible to make a value judgment as far as kinoart, or any kind of art, is concerned. People will prefer different patterns because each person has a unique frame of reference that is based on (1) the way the brain selects and organizes sensations into meaningful patterns, and (2) the brain's storage of memories, associations, and emotions.

Other Factors

In addition to the factors already discussed, many others affect the way a person perceives an event. For instance, the meaning or feeling a person attaches to a sensation depends, in part, on the situation. When a man is relaxing in the glow of a crackling fireplace with a liberating libation and a special lady, the aroma of burning wood will enhance his contentment. However, if the same man is awakened in the middle of the night by the smell of burning wood, the emotions aroused will be anxiety and fright.

The circumstances of a situation also affect kinesthetic perceptions. If you're new to the sport of bodybuilding and attempt to lift maximal weight, it's extremely doubtful you will enjoy the associated body music. Deep within the brain a tiny voice will be muttering something like, "Hey fool, you're just asking for a hernia." On the other hand, if you've been training for years, the intense sensations produced by maximal exertions may inspire the brain to sigh, "Oo-o that feels good. Do it again. Do it again."

Memories, too, will accent the perceptions associated with body music. Because of interconnections between memory circuits in the brain, people associate sensations with related events, things, or people. If the experiences are pleasant, the sensations will tend to be perceived in a positive way.

A personal illustration occurred recently when my wife brought home a box of ginger snaps. It was the first time I had smelled the goodies in about 50 years. Immediately I thought of my sweet old grandma who used to give them to my twin brother and me when we were well-behaved. We didn't deserve them very often, but as I recall we always got them anyway. Grandmothers are like that, you know.

Now consider a dancer as he practices *grande jetés.* The body music of his spectacular leaps may summon memories of other *grande jetés,* perhaps a ballet in which he danced particularly well. Other memories may be the inspiring, beautiful accompanying music, resplendent costumes, a lovely prima ballerina, and an appreciative audience. All of these associations, even if they are subliminal, will enhance the dancer's perceptions of his rehearsal and of his body's music.

Associations are not limited to the past. They also apply to the present. And they may be negative as well as positive. Imagine kinoartists practicing in a dark, dingy gym where their noses are assaulted by stale sweat and their ears beleaguered by banging radiators, jangling phones, and raucous music. People may experience some pleasant kinesthesia, but it is not likely to be bolstered by the environment.

Relatively few of these gyms are still operating. A more realistic view is the modern exercise studio where patrons are pampered with soft music, scented air, thick carpets, and expensive decor. For most people these accompanying associations do have a positive effect on their exercise.

There is a fly in the ointment of modern exercise emporiums, however. Every sense is taken into consideration except one—the main one—kinesthesia. If the emphasis is not on developing the joys of body music, clients, in essence, are still "working out." They are just doing it in a pleasant environment. The medicine of exercise merely has a sugar coating. No wonder there is a high dropout rate in commercial exercise programs. Even sweet-tasting medicine becomes tiresome.

Kinoartists do not need exercise "sweeteners" because they do not perceive themselves as working out. They kinesthetically indulge themselves in the euphoric and creative aspects of physical activity. This method is far more likely to spur a lifetime of participation because people will always find time to do things that "turn them on."

This chapter has attempted to give you some insight into the vast potential of your perceptual abilities and how you can expand and control them. So armed, you can confidently embark on a kinoartistic adventure knowing the destination actually does exist and is reachable. And what is the ultimate destination of kinoart? Quite simply, it is personal fulfillment through physical activity and esthetics.

THE MEANING OF ART

4

People involved in any type of art must have some knowledge of esthetics—of what it is that makes art beautiful. Not all artists will agree with prevailing ideas, but the ideas will at least provide an intellectual starting point for their own form of art. This chapter is devoted to helping you understand and apply esthetics to your kinoart.

Such assistance is not unusual. Even for the traditional arts, classes have long been taught to help people learn what is esthetically pleasing. There are classes in painting, sculpture, architecture, and music appreciation as well as in literature. There is even a book entitled *The Art of Watching Films.* Guidance is particularly essential in this new art involving kinesthesia because it is not yet an established art form.

Some people, solely by knee-jerk reaction, will resist accepting kinoart as a bona fide artistic endeavor. As Thomas Munro, the art critic, so aptly wrote in *The Arts and Their Interrelationships:*

> *It is not easy to escape from the grooves of thought and action marked out by past authorities. It is not easy for an individual worker to establish a new terminology, a new set of theoretical distinctions in a complex field, or to make others understand them.*

There's always been resistance to new concepts—even in such established arts as painting and sculpture. The formidable French Academy of Fine Arts ostracized the impressionistic painters when they introduced their style in the 1860s. One critic said:

> *They take canvas, paint, and brushes, splash on a few colors haphazardly and sign their names to the whole.*

The sculptor Rodin was even more vehemently insulted. As late as 1916, when the sculptor had finally attained fame, a speaker in the French Senate brayed:

> *What really is this Mr. Rodin and what is his art? Demented, hallucinated, possessed, convulsive, or a humbug, Mr. Rodin claims to have enriched and even renewed art. It is a rebellion against form, order, balance, against reason and tradition, against good taste and common sense.*

Rodin, of course, eventually became widely recognized as one of the greatest sculptors in history.

More recently, when the Beatles first came to the United States, the *New York Times* described them as "asexual and homely." (That opinion, of course, was quickly overturned by hordes of female admirers.) The harm in such knee-jerk reactions, especially by salaried critics, is that many people will blindly believe them and thereby be deprived of much pleasure.

Before a general definition of art is offered here, it must be recognized that art in its broadest interpretation can include practically every action and product of humanity. The term "art" in such a context would have very little meaning. And maybe that's not a bad situation. In Bali, for instance, there's no word in their language for "art." Yet, it's impossible to imagine a culture where art is such an integral part of everyday life. In Bali, life *is* art. Because art enhances our pleasure, perhaps it's no coincidence that the Balinese are thought by many to be the happiest people on earth.

Art is not nearly as pervasive in Europe and America as it is in Bali. Here and across the Atlantic, art is set aside in its own niche. As such, it's little wonder the Western cultures have established limits in their definitions of art. This book is not going to attempt to change this limiting attitude (that would be a highly unrealistic undertaking.) However, it must be said that narrow definitions of art do restrict an artist's creativity.

As might be expected, this range of beliefs explains why after thousands of years of interpretation, there is still no single definition of art that will satisfy everyone. As Beethoven wrote in 1810:

> *Art! Who comprehends her? With whom can one consult concerning this great goddess? The answer might be, "We can at least try to understand the goddess."*

Yes, we can try. But defining art is difficult because it is such a personal matter. Whether an object or event is art depends, in part, on the intentions of the artist. It also depends on the opinion of a spectator. An artist and spectator, of course, may disagree on whether a work should be called art. Fortunately, this problem is eliminated in kinoart because the participant is simultaneously both the artist and the spectator.

With these reservations in mind, the definition of art presented in Chapter One is again stated. Namely, art refers to those objects and events which (1) are *perceived* through the senses, (2) are organized toward a *unified experience,* and (3) result in an *esthetic event.* Although simply stated, much is implied in these three criteria.

As shown previously, kinoart can be *perceived* through the kinesthetic sense. That satisfies the first criteria. Evidence has also been given to show the importance of the kinesthetic sense and its potential richness. Of course, because perceptions vary according to an individual's interests, personality, philosophy, and so on, it follows that no matter how identical the kinesthesia, each person will perceive the patterns differently. Further, few people will organize their kinesthetic sensations into the unified experiences required for art, except through training.

Although nature provides the raw material for art and may itself be esthetically appealing, it tends to be exceedingly complex, profuse, and disorganized. As a result, the effect is often a meaningless and unpleasant jumble of sensations.

A purely physiological analogy to this phenomenon is the prickly sensation you feel in your arm or hand when you lie on it the wrong way. The limb goes to sleep because the blood flow to it is cut off. That deprivation starves the nerves. As a result, the nerve impulses to the brain become so chaotic that the brain interprets them as meaningless static.

A jumble of sensations helps to explain why the kinesthesia of exercise can be overlooked—or worse, thought to be unpleasant. The excessive variety and disorganization of the sensations can make them meaningless and sometimes even irritating, like static on a radio. This kinesthetic static may be the reason so many people find exercising unpleasant. Bringing order to nature's swirl of sensations is where the artist steps in. To quote Aristotle:

> *Art completes what nature cannot bring to a finish. The artist gives us [and himself] a knowledge of nature's unrealized ends.*

Kinoartists do this by skillfully choosing, limiting, and emphasizing various sensations as they organize them into *unified experiences* that are easier to comprehend.

The phrase, "easier to understand," should give relief to people who believe I am implying that art surpasses nature. Art surpass nature? No, that is inconceivable. Perhaps human beings just don't have the capacity to see the completeness of nature. It's difficult for anyone to disagree with Sir Thomas Browne's statement (Religio Medici, sec. 16):

> *Nature is the art of God.*

What is being suggested here is that an artist organizes and simplifies the complexities of nature so the simple minds of humans can better comprehend and appreciate nature.

The organizing of a profusion of elements also applies to literature. Mark Twain explained, in his typically delightful way, when he wrote:

> *With a hundred words to do it with, the artisan could catch that airy thought and tie it down and reduce it to a . . . cabbage, but the artist does it with only twenty, and the thought is a flower.*

A down-to-earth example of disunity is a typical teenager's room. Some might claim the room is an interior decorator's version of Jackson Pollock's painting, *Autumn Rhythm.*

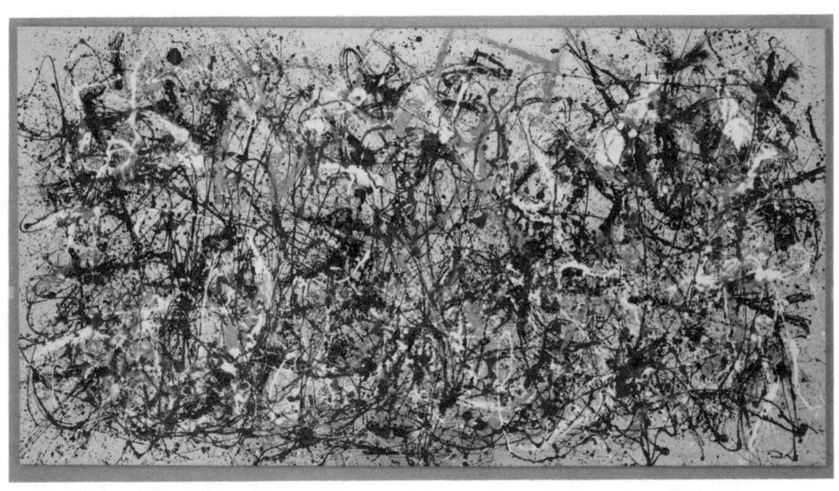

Fig. 4-1. Jackson Pollock. *Autumn Rhythm.* The Metropolitan Museum of Art, George A. Hearn Fund, 1957. New York.

Mothers, who seem to be natural artists, periodically make forays into such a chamber and skillfully select which articles must be eliminated and then organize the remaining in closets, drawers, shelves, and bookcases. The result is an esthetically appealing pattern which has been known to persist, in rare cases, for as long as an hour.

Similarly, your brain can take the superabundant kinesthetic sensations that gush into it during physical activity, and by careful selection, organize the sensations according to characteristics such as quality, intensity, location, duration, and rhythm. Your brain can do this organization by concentrating on some sensations, thus magnifying their intensities—and ignoring others, thus diminishing their intensities. With virtuosity, achieved only through practice, a kinesthetic pattern is created with each element meaningfully relating to others, making a unified experience.

You can depend solely on your brain's ability to deal with the kinesthetic sensations. However, the results are likely to be far more esthetic if you plan and control the sensations. This is done simply by controlling the movement of your joints and the tension in your muscles.

Your body music can become a unified experience much like that of a painting. The difference is that a painter creates a unified design of visual sensations while a kinoartist creates one of kinesthetic sensations—but both works of art are expressions of the artists's thoughts and emotions.

A work of art is far more than just a unified experience, though. The experience must be an esthetic event. Or, as most definitions of art declare, art must be beautiful. And this makes sense as long as one realizes that beauty is not necessarily akin to the prettiness exemplified by Renoir's *Portrait of a Young Girl.* As a matter of fact, many masterpieces portray ugliness or repulsion. Examples are Goya's painting *Saturn Devouring His Children,* Shakespeare's play *Macbeth,* and Poe's short story *The Masque of the Red Death.*

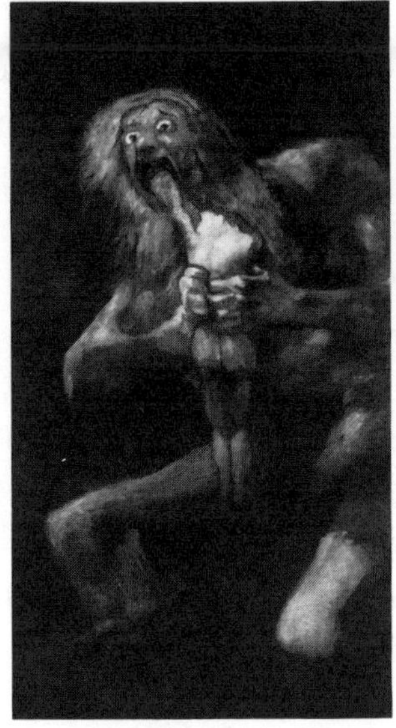

Saturn Devouring His Children
Francisco Goya. 1819-23
The Prado Museum, Madrid.

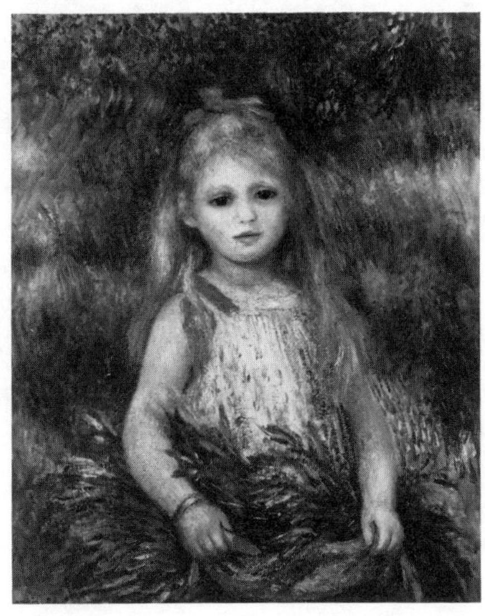

Fig. 4-2. "Beauty is Truth."
Portrait of a Young Girl
Pierre Auguste Renoir
(limoges, 1841 - Cagnes, Nice 1919)
Menina com as espigas
Col. Museu de Arte
de Saõ Paulo Assis Chateaubriand.

Photo: Luiz Hossaka

It's easy to understand why we enjoy art that is graceful, lovely, and harmonious. But what is the attraction of art that is harsh, discordant, or sordidly realistic. The standard explanation is that all of these characteristics are part of the human experience. And an accurate representation of any such characteristic, whether physical, intellectual, or emotional, can be considered beautiful. That is what Keats had in mind when he wrote:

Beauty is truth, truth beauty

The attraction of unpretty works of art suggests that an artist should consider creating a broad range of esthetic experiences including the "unpretty" along with the "pretty." A comparison of Goya's *Clothed Maja* with his *Saturn* shows such variability by an artist is possible. Indeed, the stretching of one's talents and imagination is the essential quality of an artist.

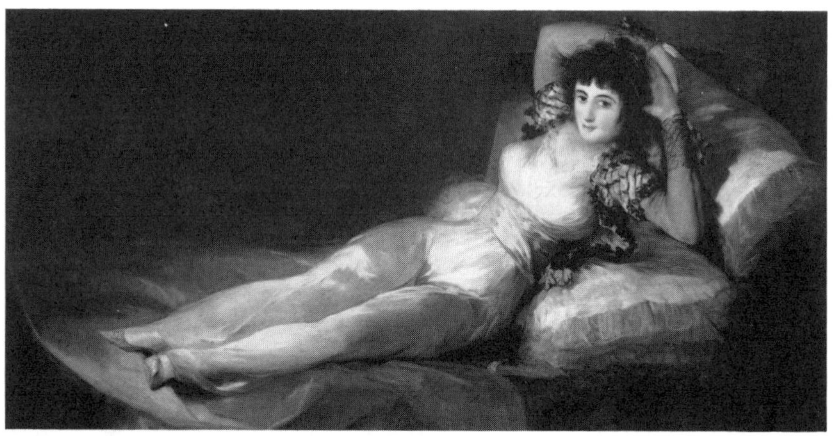

Fig. 4-3. Francisco Goya. *The Clothed Maja.* 1800. Museo del Prado, Madrid.

As a kinoartist, you should strive to arrange your kinesthesia into patterns that are esthetic experiences. Even more, you should continually expand your body music repertoire to include not only smooth, graceful, and "pretty" movements, but ones that are disrhythmic, jerky, and intense, even painful. These unpretty sensations can also be perceived as interestingly honest, that is, beautiful.

Can pain be pleasurable? Though the thought seems paradoxical, it is not original. Bayard Taylor stated:

> *There's a pang in all rejoicing, a joy in the heart of pain.*

The sentiment was stated with even greater brevity by Ralph Waldo Emerson:

> *Under pain, pleasure—under pleasure, pain lies.*

A top female bodybuilder in the 1980s, Stacey Bentley, applied the idea to exercise when she declared that she exercised even when she did not feel like doing it. She said there was pleasure in the pain—that it "blew her mind." Many athletes express similar feelings.

It may be amusing to hear athletes speak of the beauty and joy they experienced during their event when their faces were contorted in agony. But such struggles are moments of truth and, again, truth is beauty.

Yes, kinoartists should occasionally use sensations of pain in their works of art—not the pain of injury, but the pain of intense effort and the lactic acid it produces. Still, heroic physical exertions and powerful emotions are not necessary to produce kinoart. Everyone creates kinoart everyday, almost constantly, in fact. They are simply not aware of it, just as children who are leaping and skipping and pirouetting do not realize they are dancing.

Physical activity is a large part of nearly every person's life—not just exercise programs but all forms of movement. Such activities have the potential to be artistic expressions—or more specifically to be kinoart. A modest example presented earlier in this book is a yawn. Yawn again and concentrate on the sensations. As your muscles contract and stretch, you will (1) clearly perceive the sensations of kinesthesia, (2) notice the sensations are organized into a unified pattern that is recognized as a yawn and (3) find the experience a pleasant one. Here, all the criteria of art being met by a simple yawn—if you concentrate on the kinesthesia.

The next time you yawn, make a conscious effort to exaggerate the act. There are no limitations. You may even want to vocalize, using whining sounds, screams, or Tarzan yodels. The sounds will only enhance the total sensual, intellectual, and emotional experience of the kinoart. It might be a good idea, however, to do this when there are no strangers nearby.

I like to accompany my wake-up yawn in the morning an earth-shattering roar pirated from the "king of the jungle." While vocalizing, I stretch my powerful muscles and shake my tawny mane, or more precisely, my gray mane. And to be completely candid, I suppose it's a tad too thin to be considered a mane.

Vocalizations are not unusual in exercise sessions and sporting events. Anyone who has visited a bodybuilding gymnasium would agree. Similarly, the screaming "kiai" is an integral part of karate. Even in professional tennis, that traditional bastion of gentility, spectators are often treated to dramatic vocal displays by players.

Yawns are not unique sources of kinesthetic pleasure. The kinesthesia of every physical activity can become body music. Some activities may not be especially "artistic" or satisfying at first, but with practice, you will become more and more adept at selecting and organizing your kinesthetic sensations so they *will* become more and more pleasing.

Why not make the effort? As McCarter and Gilbert state in *Living with Art:*

> *We can go through life like sleepwalkers, ignoring or taking for granted the art around [and within] us. Or we can enrich our lives by developing a more active appreciation of the art we live with. . . . When we appreciate art we are only following a basic esthetic impulse—an urge to respond to that which is beautiful.*

The authors were writing primarily about the visual arts, but the ideas apply just as powerfully to kinoart. In fact, if art takes us places we have not been before, kinoart may well lead the artistic pack into undreamed of territories.

Kinoartists would seem to be unique among artists because they cannot directly communicate with others through their artistic works. After all, kinesthesia resides entirely within the body. That does not make kinoart any less an art than the more established ones, though. To think so would be like saying an esthetic experience produced in private by a dancer or musician is automatically less beautiful than one performed in front of an audience.

At one time modern people were unaware of the art made by prehistoric cave men (or women), but that certainly did not mean those primitive cultures did not produce art. And it doesn't mean the primitive works magically became art upon their discovery. Similarly, the poems of Emily Dickinson did not suddenly become works of art (*voilá*) upon their publication after her death; they were just as artistic when she lifted her pen from the page as when they were discovered years later.

Indeed, it can be argued that all art occurs and exists solely in an artist's imagination; and paintings, musical scores, and dance compositions are merely imperfect manifestations of the art. Spectators, then, can experience these manifestations, these works of art, but not the art itself which is locked in the imagination of each artist.

We can all be artists and take pleasure from activities such as painting, music, and kinoart. We don't have to be especially proficient, as long as we enjoy ourselves. It is the *striving* to have beauty in our lives that makes for a more fulfilling, happier life. The painter, Thomas Hart Benton, wrote:

The only way an artist can fail is to quit work.

But there is a more fundamental way for an artist to fail; it is by not starting. It would be a shame to deprive yourself of the joys of body music merely because you do not start. The shame is magnified because involvement in the medium of kinoart is so easy.

PUTTING FORM IN KINOART

5

Art appreciation is a combination of intuitive enjoyment and an understanding of esthetics. You're much more likely to enjoy art you understand. Conversely, the more you understand art, the more you'll enjoy it. As an aspiring kinoartist, you must therefore learn what makes art desirable or undesirable. This is most efficiently done by understanding the laws of esthetics.

True, there are no *absolute* laws for determining artistic values. But there are some common elements in a work of art that people generally find pleasing. These principles are not so much laws as they are guidelines, but they have at least placed artistic creation and evaluation on a fairly objective basis.

A wise application of the laws of esthetics will greatly help you create and appreciate your body music. At the same time, particularly as you become more experienced, you should not so slavishly follow these guidelines that they limit your kinesthetic expression. After all, the laws for determining what is artistic are not binding or precise.

The principles of esthetics can be divided into two groups. The first is the *form* of a work of art and the other is its intellectual and emotional *content.*

Form is the way the elements are organized in a work of art. In violin playing, the elements are the sounds that are produced. In kinoart (body music), the elements of form are the kinesthetic sensations.

For ease of discussion, however, when planning a kinoartistic experience, the movements and tensions themselves may be thought of as the elements of form. Activities ranging from the lifting of an eyebrow to a competitive ice skating routine may be considered body music—as long as people realize the real work of art comes from the kinesthesia produced by those activities. Therefore, above all, kinoartists must concentrate on their kinesthetic sensations.

There are two ways to control the form of your art. You can vary either its *design* or its *pattern,* or both. Admittedly, not everyone will agree with this categorization, but there is not a lot of agreement on any aspect of art. Most of the controversies have to do with terminology and organization, though. The basic beliefs are usually not strikingly different.

The system presented here has been chosen simply for the ease with which it can be applied to kinoart. As used here, design puts variety in a movement or exercise session. Pattern has the opposite function. It ties elements together to instill order or unity.

In discussing esthetics, musical examples are the most appropriate comparison to kinoart since the two art forms have so many characteristics in common. For instance, both kinoart and music have easily perceived rhythms, frequency, and intensity variations. The only difference is that music consists of sound sensations and kinoart consists of kinesthetic sensations.

As you know by now, kinesthesia can be considered the body's music. If each of the body's 600 muscles is an individual instrument, it's easy to think of the body as a large symphony. What's difficult to imagine, though, is the marvelous range, depth, and nuances of the body's kinesthetic music. And remember, there are about 200 joints in the body. Each movement can vary in direction, magnitude, and the pressure exerted on the joint. All of these variations create different sensations. You can see that the size of the symphony is almost beyond comprehension. But you are the conductor and can "play" an infinite number of kinoartistic pieces.

In spite of the close similarities between kinoart and music, visual examples are generally used in this chapter to help you understand esthetics and apply it to kinoart. There are several reasons for doing so. In the first place, because we are so strongly oriented to the visual sense, we tend to learn more easily in that sensory system. Besides, it's nearly as difficult to capture the qualities of sound on paper as it is for kinesthesia. In truth, it cannot be done for either sense, but visual symbols *can* represent kinesthetic sensations.

Design

Any work of art that is boring is a disaster. Design techniques help to avoid that by using contrast, gradation, theme-and-variation, and restraint. Contrast is the simplest and most striking technique. One way to achieve contrast in kinoart is by varying joint movements and the tension in muscles.

Imagine a social dance in which a couple continually walks in a straight line. Not only would a very long dance floor be required, the kinesthesia would be monotonous due to a lack of contrasts. A waltz is different. Instead of a series of identical steps, a waltz consists of steps that vary in length, time, and direction. Because of these contrasts, a single waltz pattern (such as a box step), even when performed over and over, is far more pleasing, kinesthetically, than regular walking. Of course, even the waltz box step tends to become kinesthetically boring after awhile. To prevent this a couple can use a variety of waltz patterns to increase the number of contrasts.

You have to be careful, though. If a work of art contains more than four or five *unrelated* contrasts, the work starts to become confusing. Confusion can be reduced or eliminated, however, by choosing contrasts that are related either by gradation or theme-and-variation techniques.

A waltz, for instance, may consist of many stepping patterns and still not be confusing because each pattern is a variation of the same rhythm—ONE, two, three; ONE, two, three; etc. Because the variations are related, there is a unity that reduces confusion.

This theme-and-variation method is especially useful in keeping complex activities, such as sports, from becoming kinesthetically confusing. While each sport contains many movement contrasts, there are unifying relationships in each. A tennis player, for example, will make hundreds of strokes during a match. If each stroke was an unrelated contrast, the game would be very confusing—not just in learning and playing it, but also as a kinoartistic experience. The strokes, however, are not completely different. Each is just a variation of a theme, which instructors should stress.

For a typical player that theme pertains to the biomechanics of each stroke, which are essentially the same for all strokes. More specifically, the laws of biomechanics relate to balance and forces. These relatively few laws not only apply to all tennis strokes—they apply to all physical activities. If your movements are biomechanically sound, your body music will tend to be satisfying. While the biomechanical theme keeps the strokes from becoming confusing, there will be enough variation between strokes to keep the game from becoming boring.

A tennis game, admittedly, will be confusing to beginning players. They execute each stroke so differently there can be little perceived relatedness in either biomechanics or kinesthesia. As they continue to practice, though, players will gradually become aware of the similarities between strokes. When they see that each stroke is just a variation of a theme, the confusion will disappear and their game will rapidly improve and be a lot more satisfying.

Confusion in art can also be reduced by choosing contrasts that gradually change. A visual example of gradation is a sequence of gray shapes ranging from light to dark. Fig. 5-1 shows how such a gradation (A) compares with six shapes arranged in no particular order as in (B). Notice, the gradation in (A) exists not only in intensity, but in shapes and spacing. The gradation, very clearly, results in a sense of order. This is not to say, however, that pattern (A) is an esthetically more pleasing design than (B). That determination is an individual judgment, but (A) is clearly more orderly and harmonious.

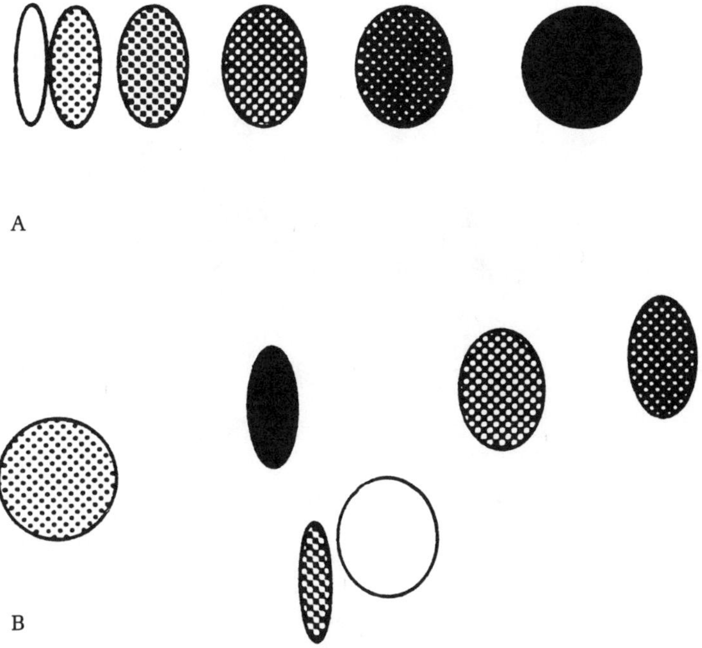

Fig. 5-1. Gradation Related Contrasts (A) versus Unrelated Contrasts (B).

A kinesthetic example of gradation is demonstrated in Fig. 5-2 by a woman doing arm curls with dumbbells. She is creating kinoart by concentrating on her kinesthesia as she performs six arm curl repetitions. Even though the weight remains the same, the tension she feels in her biceps increases with each repetition due to fatigue. In other words, each repetition contrasts with the others. But even though there are six contrasts, there's not even a hint of confusion in the body music because the contrasts are related. In this case, the contrasts have to do with the gradual increase in muscular tension.

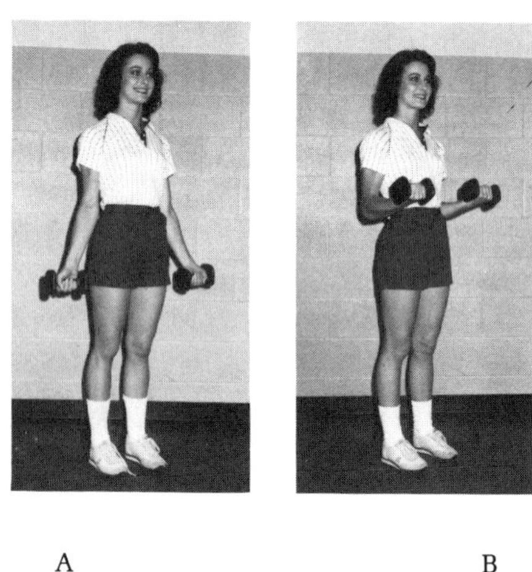

A B

Fig. 5-2. An Arm Curl Exercise (A repetition consists of lifting the weights from position "A" to "B" and returning them to "A").

This set of arm curls also has the esthetically desirable characteristic of *climax.* As each repetition progressively requires more effort, it engages the woman's attention more forcefully until her kinesthetic awareness reaches its climax during the final repetition. A literary example of climax may best be seen in a mystery story. To maintain reader interest the tension must increase throughout the story and reach its climax at the end.

Kinesthetic gradations can be created in many ways other than number. A common method is to vary movement. One of the many possibilities is to lift a barbell just a short distance with the first curling motion and then lift it a little higher with each succeeding repetition. The climax for movement, as well as tension, will be when the weight is curled all the way up on the last repetition.

The techniques of contrast, gradation, and theme-and-variation help to prevent exercise sessions from becoming monotonous at one extreme and confusing at the other—that is, they keep exercise sessions kinesthetically interesting. Interest, however, can itself become tiresome.

The purpose of the *restraint* technique is to prevent this waning effect from occurring. The technique merely involves relaxing between periods of tension (or movement). The reasoning is that after a period of relaxation, even a brief one, a person returns to an activity with renewed interest. Relaxation can occur either with complete rest or an activity that's not as interesting.

The bar graph in Fig. 5-3 pertains to softball, but it can be used just as well to represent the body music of the woman's six arm curls where each curl requires a progressive increase of the tension in her biceps. The spaces in-between the bars indicate periods of relaxation (restraint) that keep the woman's interest in her kinesthesia from diminishing.

In the illustration, you can see that all the techniques of design are used; contrast for variety, theme-and-variation and gradation to reduce confusion, and restraint to keep interest from diminishing. Notice that the climax occurs at the end of the set just before a long period of relaxation begins.

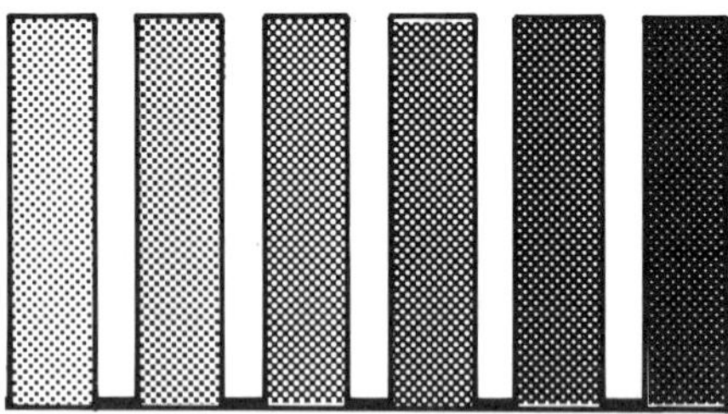

Fig. 5-3. The Kinesthetic (or Emotional) Interest of a Softball Batter as He:

A. walks to home plate

B. practices a swing with the bat

C. checks his swing on the first pitch

D. fouls off the second pitch

E. safely hits the third pitch for a single

F. runs to first base

(The increasingly darkened bars represent periods of increased interest. The spaces in-between represent periods of restraint or relaxation.)

Not every trip to the plate will be an esthetically satisfying kinesthetic experience. The batter may just stand at the plate and let the pitcher throw three strikes. In that case the coach would undoubtedly explain to the batter, "My boy, you *do* realize that was quite unappealing kinesthetically, don't you?"

Pattern

Whereas design gives interest to a work of art through variety, pattern provides order and unity through organization. This unifying process reduces confusion because a pattern has more meaning than randomly scattered elements—whether the elements are visual, auditory, or kinesthetic in nature.

The key aspect of pattern is the number of elements in a work of art. If the pattern is to be esthetically pleasing, the elements should be limited to a number that can be easily perceived. Again, this number normally lies between one and five (with eight being the maximum). Less is often more, in regards to the number of elements in a pattern.

To illustrate this, if three marbles are tossed onto a carpet as shown in Fig. 5-4, your brain will immediately perceive the group of marbles as consisting of three elements. However, if seven marbles are tossed, your brain will *not* immediately perceive the group as consisting of seven elements; you will have to count them to determine the number. Seven elements are clearly more than most people can mentally grasp with ease.

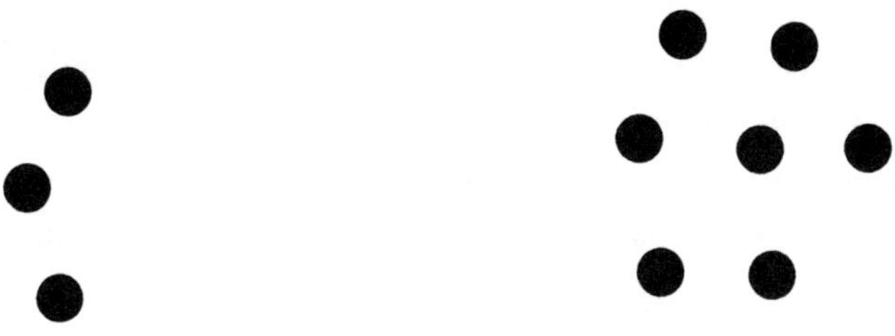

Fig. 5-4. A Three Element Group and a Seven Element Group.

Advertisers are well-aware of the average person's ability to "handle" a low number of elements. That's why a 1980s fast food commercial had an abrasive (but endearing), old woman asking a competitor, "Where's the Beef?" The three-word ad was very effective. But how effective do you think it would have been if she had asked, "Could you tell me where the beef is on this hamburger?" Or even, "Where is the beef on this burger?"

Politicians know the value of brevity. Now, I am not suggesting you adopt all the techniques and ethics of politicians. But we *can* learn some things from them. For instance, when political managers devise slogans, they (the smart ones) use as few words as possible to make the greatest impression. In 1952, Dwight Eisenhower won the presidency with "I Like Ike." In 1979, Gerald Ford's campaign slogan was simply "Win." Well, he did not win. The slogan was fine, but it was not enough to overcome some heavy negative baggage with such labels as "Nixon," "Watergate," and "Pardon."

The use of few elements can, of course, be applied to exercise. For proof, have a person do repetitions (reps) of any exercise, say, arm curls. Have him try not to count. After he has done 12 reps, ask him how many he has done. He will not know because the number is too high to be easily perceived. Ask the same question after six reps, though, and the chances are much greater that he will know. And if you ask the same question after three reps, he will know for sure. Three is a number that is easily perceived, intellectually and kinesthetically. It's that ease of perception that makes the associated body music less confusing and, therefore, more pleasant for people who find exercise boring.

As stated in Chapter Three, the brain automatically organizes stimuli into groups to give them more meaning. One person will organize stimuli one way and another person may do it a different way due to chance or differences in genetic or cultural backgrounds. As a result, one person may divide the large group of seven marbles into smaller groups as shown in Fig. 5-5 (A), while another might do so as in (B). Both people will, by coincidence, have organized the seven elements into a pattern consisting of three groups. Each group thereby becomes an element itself—a complex element, but still an element. And three elements is a number that most people can easily grasp mentally.

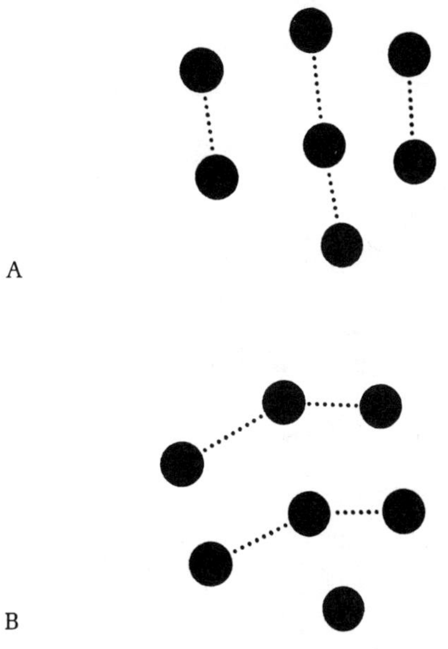

Fig. 5-5. Two Ways in Which a Person Might Organize Seven Elements into Three Groups.

Let's assume the two people in the previous example did not consciously organize the marbles into a pattern. That is, the organizations occurred automatically—or subjectively. In such cases, whether the visual patterns will be pleasing is strictly hit or miss. They are just as likely to be confusing and unpleasing.

The value of planning is demonstrated in Fig. 5-6. In (A) the crescent-shaped elements are distributed randomly, and viewers are left to subjectively organize the elements into patterns as they see fit. In (B) a Viking artist many years ago organized the identical elements into a pattern whose form is perceived in the way the artist intended. Because of the planning by the artist, the six random elements have been arranged into a pattern that, in essence, becomes a single, complex element. Since the pattern is easily perceived as a single element, it is not confusing to the viewer. Clearly, the organized elements are more satisfying to the average eye than the haphazardly arranged elements.

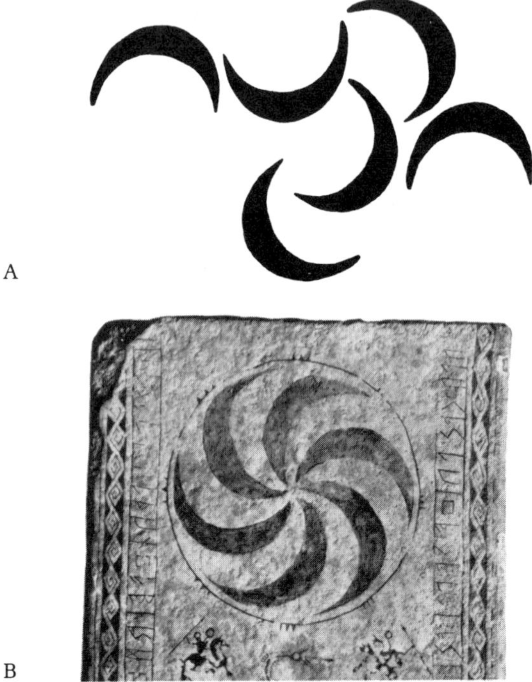

Fig. 5-6. Six Crescent-Shaped Elements Arranged Randomly (A) and Organized into a Pattern by a Viking Artist (B). Picture-Stone from Martebo, Gotland, Sweden. 5th to 7th Cent. A.T.A., Stockholm.

Skillful planning of physical activity is also likely to produce more satisfying sensations of movement than those of unplanned movements. Imagine an exercise session consisting of one arm curl, three knee bends, three push-ups, one knee bend, three arm curls, one push-up, three arm curls, one push-up, two knee bends, and one push-up. It's difficult to perceive a pattern in this ungrouped movements. Not only will there be kinesthetic confusion, there will be intellectual confusion—you will nearly always lose track of the number of repetitions of each movement. Even seeing the program on paper is confusing. To give order to the kinesthesia, you can simply perform all six arm curls consecutively, then six knee bends, and finally the six push-ups. This creates three easily recognized groups each consisting of six elements. Each group of six *simple* exercise elements, in essence, becomes a single *complex* element, which is analagous to the pattern on the Viking picture-stone.

Although the primary role of patterns in art is to eliminate confusion through order and unity, patterns can themselves be sources of delight if they possess rhythm. The sounds made by a tap dancer, for instance, are exciting not for the individual sounds (elements) but for the rhythmic patterns formed by them. Similarly, the individual kinesthetic sensations experienced by the tap dancer are not nearly so captivating as the rhythmic kinesthetic patterns.

The beginning of mankind's (which, of course, includes womankind's) love affair with rhythm is lost in the mists of time. Further, in each individual, the romance with rhythm begins long before birth with the comforting sounds of his or her mother's heart beat. Most animals are captivated by rhythm. That's why a ticking clock will calm a motherless puppy.

Humans are unique, though, because they apparently are the only animals who consciously control rhythm. This is observed in virtually every culture in visual designs as well as in sound and movement. Rhythm is an important aspect of all art from poetry (where it is referred to as meter) to architecture. The repetition of the windows in Fig. 5-7 illustrates a beat as regular as a metronome's.

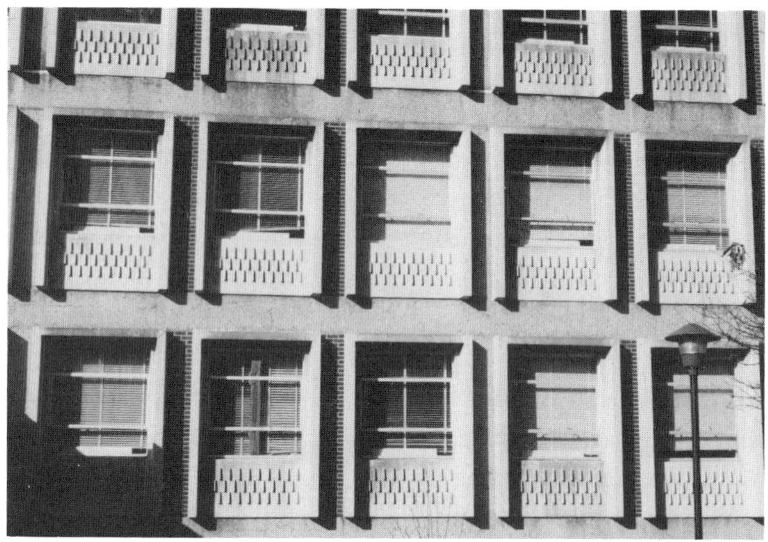

Fig. 5-7. Series of Windows, Mitchell Hall (University of Memphis). 1993.

The simplest patterns are called *elementary* patterns. They should consist of eight or fewer elements. An example of an elementary kinesthetic pattern is a series of six vertical hops with each hop being very similar. Another elementary pattern is a set of arm curls with the repetitions equally paced. Elements that make-up an elementary pattern can also be dissimilar. That occurs, for example, in a ballroom dance (say, a fox trot) where many different steps may be used.

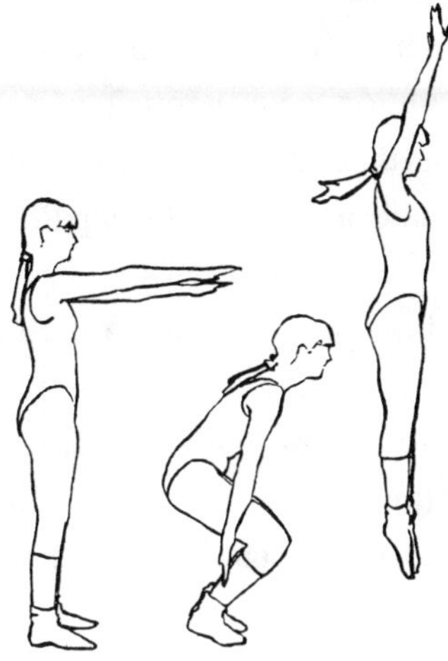

Fig. 5-8. Vertical Hops.

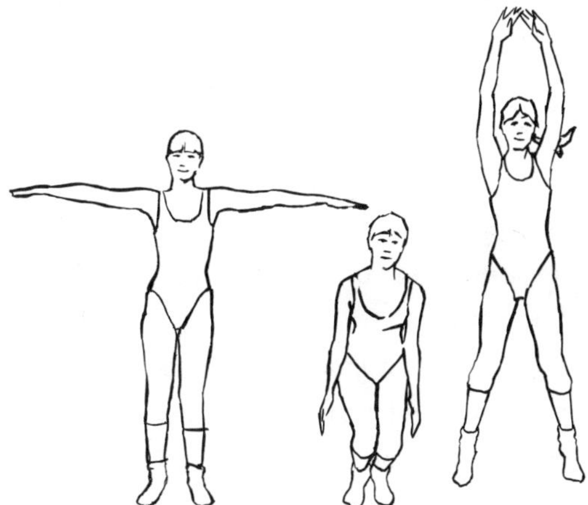

Fig. 5-9. Side-Straddle Hops.

The woman in Fig. 5-8 can create *quantitative* differences by varying the height of her hops. The differences in the strength of muscular contractions, of course, results in differences in the kinesthetic feelings of each element.

An elementary pattern can also have *qualitative* variations in its elements. Just as a high frequency musical note is qualitatively different than a low note, the body music of a side-straddle hop is qualitatively different than a vertical hop. A person can use both types of hops to create an elementary pattern with dissimilar quality elements.

Once you know how to create elementary patterns, combination patterns are the next step. They are created by combining elementary ones. That's accomplished by either extending elementary patterns or by superimposing one upon another.

The simplest way to extend an elementary pattern is to repeat it. Because a set of eight push-ups is an elementary pattern, a simple combination pattern is formed by doing two or more sets of the push-ups with a rest period between sets.

A baseball player produces the same type of repetitive pattern during batting practice. Each swing of the bat may be considered an elementary movement pattern—its kinesthetic elements are the individual joint movements and muscular tensions associated with the swing. A basketball player practicing free throws and a ballet dancer practicing *tour jetés* are also creating repetitive movements. If these athletes *concentrate* on their body music, they will also experience kinesthetic patterns.

Non-repetitive elementary patterns are also possible. Common examples are seen in athletic games. A basketball game, for instance, consists of a non-repetitive series of dribbling, passing, and shooting patterns. Because of their diversity, a series of non-repetitive patterns is kinesthetically more interesting than a series of repetitious ones. This is one reason why many people enjoy "shooting baskets" more than lifting weights.

By superimposing one kinesthetic pattern on another, you can create interesting combinations. Consider Fig. 5-10 and the body music experienced by a person while he is riding a rollaboard (A) and while he is juggling three clubs (B). A far more complicated and exciting kinesthetic pattern results when he superimposes the juggling pattern upon the rollaboard pattern (C).

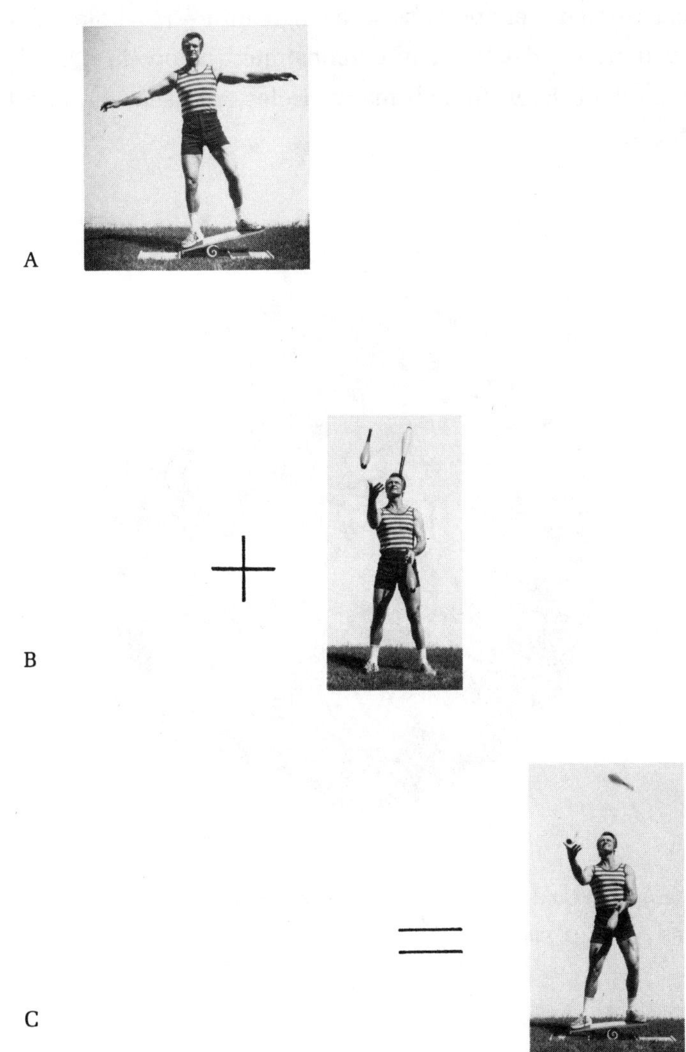

Fig. 5-10. Superimposing the Pattern of Juggling on that of Rollaboarding.

When the number of combination patterns becomes too large to be pleasing, generally more than five, you can simply organize them into structures called systems. In other words, combination patterns can be organized into a larger, orderly pattern which one can immediately perceive as a single unit—a "whole." The use of systems in visual art is demonstrated below in a gold Viking ornament. Even though many circles are used, the effect is not confusing.

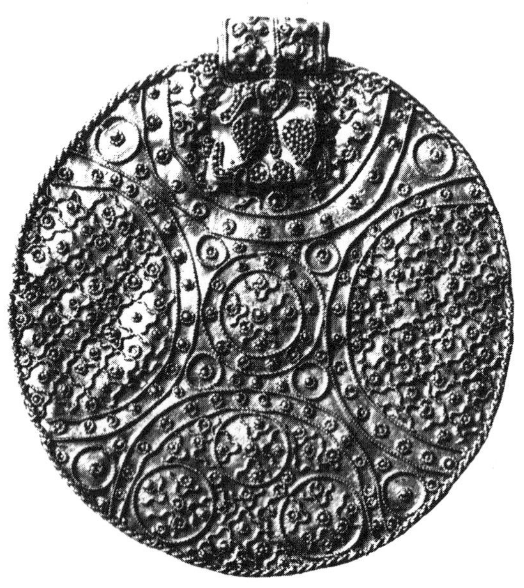

Fig. 5-11. A Gold Viking Clothing Accessory with an Artistic System of Circles. 865 - 925 A.D. Statens Historiska Museum, Stockholm.

A comparable system for the kinoartist is a typical weight training program. Each repetition of an exercise can be considered an element. Each set of repetitions forms an elementary pattern. Three sets of a particular exercise, such as the bench press, make up an extended combination pattern. Finally, a training session consisting of three sets of ten different exercises creates a system. Because of this organization, a person perceives his or her training session as orderly and comprehensible—instead of chaotic. Similar organization is also used in dance classes and practice sessions for such sports as football, baseball, and karate. For all these activities to be perceived as body music, though, people have to *concentrate* on the sensations arising from their muscles and joints.

Balance

Along with rhythmic patterns, the characteristic of *balance* is one of the most important aspects to be considered in a work of art. In body music, the degree of balance can vary tremendously. Patterns may be 1) symmetrically balanced, 2) asymmetrically balanced, 3) unbalanced, or even 4) off-balanced. None is preferable to the others. Much depends on the objectives, interests, and experience of a kinoartist.

Of the four types of patterns having to do with balance, the *symmetrical* ones produce the most harmonious body music because at any instant the sensations arriving at the brain from the left and right sides of the body are nearly identical. To experience simple symmetrical kinesthesia, stand in one place and swing your arms forward and back in unison—or sit on a table and swing your legs forward and back in unison. In either case, concentrate on the sensations coming from your muscles, joints, and tendons. Far more complicated symmetrical kinesthesia results from rowing (with hands pulling in unison) or swimming with a breast stroke.

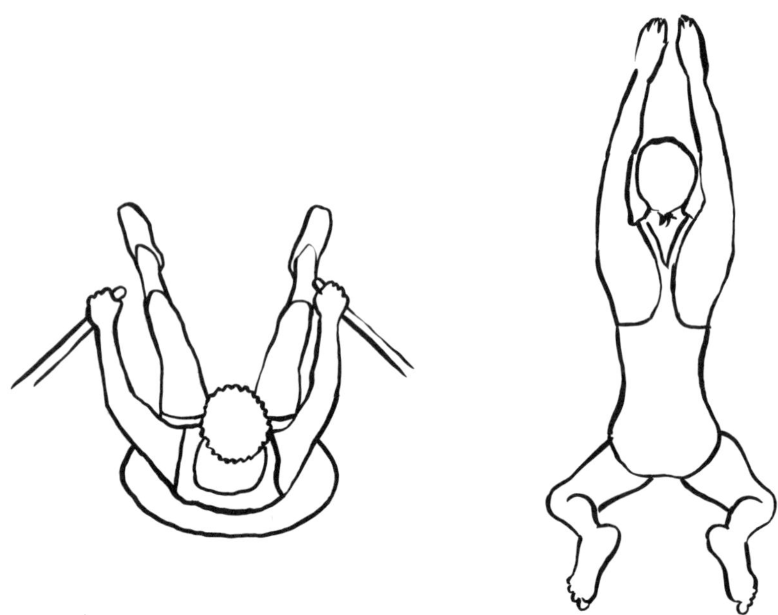

Fig. 5-12. Two Symmetrically Balanced Activities.

To experience very simple *asymmetrical* body music, stand in one place and swing your arms back and forth 180° out-of-phase as in regular walking—or sit on a table and swing your legs in a similar out-of-phase manner. The latter can also be done while sitting on the side of a swimming pool, and the sensations can be further heightened by wearing swim fins.

Asymmetrical athletic activities include rowing (with the hands simultaneously moving in opposite directions), the front crawl stroke, walking, running, biking, and skating. In all these cases the kinesthetic sensations arriving at the brain from one side of the body are 180° out-of-phase with those arriving from the other side. You'll find asymmetrical events to be less formal and more dynamic than symmetrical ones. Both kinds are usually repetitive, but there are exceptions, such as the back flip in gymnastics and the swan dive.

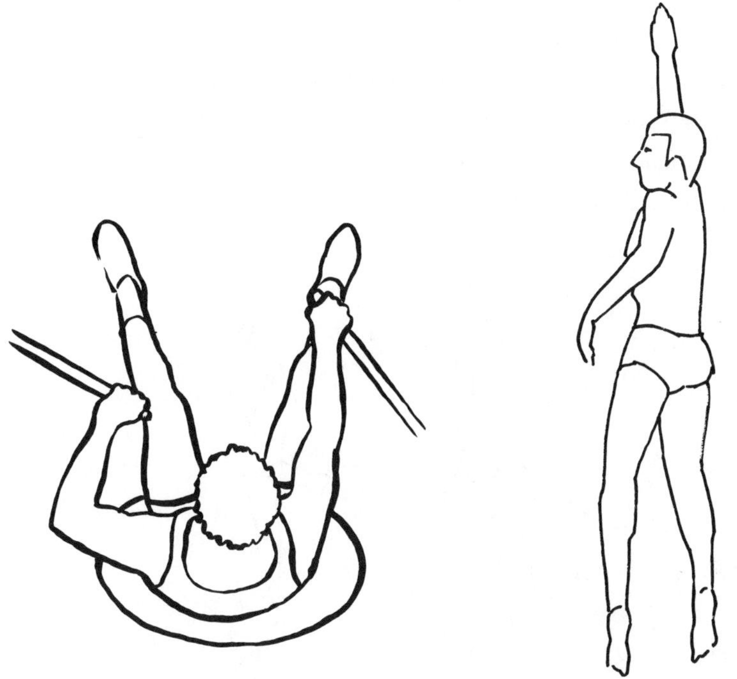

Fig. 5-13. Two Asymmetrically Balanced Activities.

In *unbalanced* activities, the kinesthetic sensations from one side of the body do not resemble those of the other side. Unbalanced patterns predominate in sports such as racquetball, basketball, and wrestling. Because these patterns are non-repetitive, they tend to be kinesthetically more interesting than activities consisting of balanced patterns.

Off-balanced kinesthetic patterns occur when a person is falling off-balance. In most of these cases equilibrium is quickly regained. Anytime you take a step, for instance, you have to first fall off-balance in the direction you wish to move before stepping off. When the foot strikes the ground, you regain your balance. Walking consists of a series of these "balanced, off-balanced" cycles. The same is true of running except that its off-balanced phase is much longer than its balanced phase. Strictly speaking, both walking and running may be described as asymmetrically off-balanced skills. Hopping forward with the feet together is a symmetrically off-balanced skill.

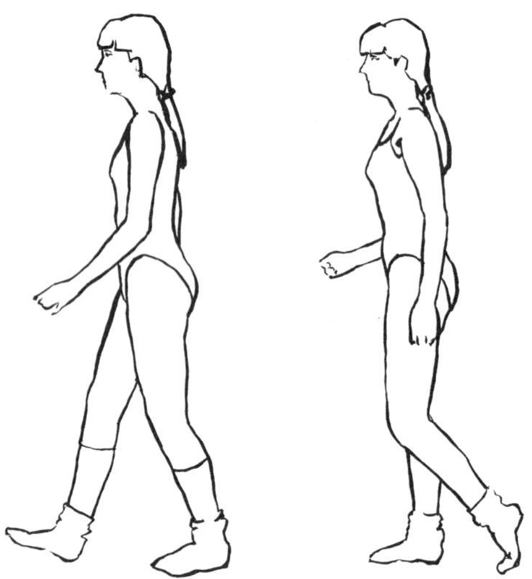

Fig. 5-14. Walking is a "Balance/Off-balance" Activity.

Rollaboarding is a far more delicate off-balance situation than either walking or running. And unicycling is probably the most fiendishly off-balanced activity yet devised. If you try it, you'll surely agree. When pedaling forward, a unicyclist is constantly off-balance—he has to be to keep moving. The trick, as shown in Fig. 5-15, is to control the degree of off-balance (B) by varying pedaling speed and/or body lean. If he gets too unbalanced (C) the unicyclist will fall forward. But if he regains his balance (A) he will stand still.

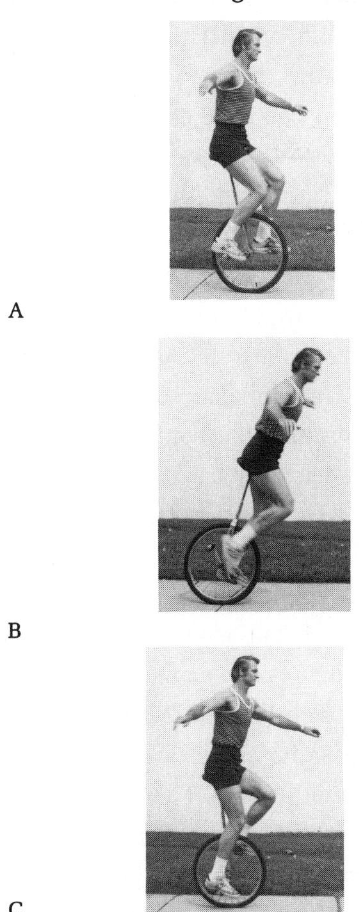

Fig. 5-15. Unicycling as an Off-Balance Activity.

People like balance because it represents order and results in a pleasant, harmonious kinoartistic experience. Conversely, as a state of unbalance increases, its effect becomes proportionately more disturbing. A visual example is a painting that hangs crookedly on a wall. The more unbalanced it is, the more jarring its effect. This concept also applies to the body music associated with off-balance physical activities.

Excessive order or balance, however, leads to boredom. For this reason, after acquiring some kinoartistic experience, you will be more appreciative of activities that are unbalanced. Although they are less orderly than their balanced counterparts, they offer more intriguing kinesthetic patterns.

Because off-balanced activities are the least orderly of all exercise patterns, they are, of course, the most exciting. The body music may be so thrilling that beginners will find the sensations unpleasant, disturbing, or even frightening.

Observe toddlers just learning to walk. As they attempt to take their first step, they panic. The off-balanced activity produces a chaotic flood of kinesthetic sensations that confuse and frighten them to the point of near paralysis. They just can't seem to take the step. This situation is not just limited to toddlers. The same phenomenon is seen in the halting attempts of an adult trying to walk a tight wire for the first time, even if the line is just a foot off the ground.

Because the orderliness of balanced patterns can become boring, off-balanced body music becomes more and more attractive. That's what finally makes children take their first step. With a bit of practice, walking loses its "wild and crazy" aspect and emerges as an exciting kinesthetic event. Then, even before walking is perfected, they are tantalized by the still more off-balanced patterns of running and, eventually, jumping, skipping, and skating. Really adventurous tykes ultimately will try to walk on their hands when they get older.

Being new to kinoart, you will probably prefer balanced kinesthetic patterns. With practice, though, you will learn to appreciate the unbalanced and off-balanced ones. You will come to enjoy all the patterns—balanced ones for their calming sense of order and off-balanced ones for provoking thrills. Indeed, as a kinoartist you should be able to devise—and relish—a wide variety of body music in design and pattern as well as balance.

PUTTING CONTENT IN KINOART

6

Art may be esthetically pleasing solely because of its form—its design, pattern, and balance. But art is far more satisfying when it has some meaning and when it arouses emotions. These intellectual and emotional facets combine to give *content* to a work of art.

Which is most important—form or content? Respected artists have trouble answering that question. Rodin himself wavered by saying:

> *Art is only feeling . . . But without the knowledge of volumes, proportions, and colors, without manual skill, the most vivid feeling is paralyzed.*

Both form and content are vital to a work of art. However, it is generally a lot harder for artists to imbue their art with content.

Some art seemingly consists solely of form. Mondrian's *Composition* (Fig. 6-1) illustrates this. A kinesthetic example is a highly structured weight training program of three sets per exercise and eight repetitions per set. Even if a work of art is based entirely on design and pattern, though, it can still have content. It's hard to imagine an artist in any medium, including kinoart, not having some reaction—either intellectual or emotional, positive or negative, to his or her creations. And it's equally difficult to imagine a viewer of art not having any reaction—positive or negative.

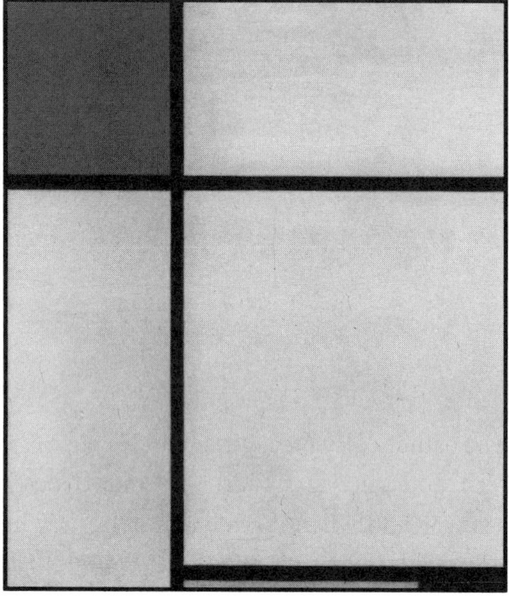

Fig. 6-1. Piet Mondrian. *Composition*. 1929. © Estate of P. Mondrian/E.M. Holtzman Trust, New York.

Intellectual Content

Intellectual content is what a work of art means or represents to either an artist or viewer. Curiosity, memory, logic, and imagination are some qualities that provide the foundation for intellectual content. However, the most important ingredient of intellectual content is probably *type*.

A type may be defined as something that is perceived as a whole even though it is made up of a group of individual characteristics. Because of this intellectual organization, type gives meaning or identity to objects and events. For instance, if you show a person a painting of a rose and ask what she sees, she'll say, "I see a rose." She will not say, "I see some red shapes clumped together, and some green, oval shapes arranged under them on a stick, and, oh yes, a lot of sharp, pointy things projecting from the stick." In other words, the individual color sensations and shapes will be perceived as a "whole"—a type. The visual type in this case is a rose.

Similarly, when swinging a softball bat, you will not perceive the movement as unrelated muscular tensions and joint movements. If you are kinesthetically aware, the action will be a single kinesthetic unit associated with the swing of a bat. The sensation of a swing is a kinesthetic type just as the rose is a visual type.

The greatest pleasure associated with a type is *recognition*. Recognition is a source of joy in most aspects of life. When you hear a long forgotten song from your youth on the radio, it will be pleasurable—even if you were not particularly fond of it originally. Similarly, most of us have been in a strange place, say a foreign city, and have crossed paths with an acquaintance. Even if you had never been very close to that person, you would be excited to see him or her. Recognition indeed brings joy.

When a baseball player hits a home run, he usually knows immediately that the ball is going out of the park from the sound and feel of contact. These sensations alone will please him, but he will be elated when he recognizes he has achieved the home run type.

A kinoartistically oriented player may also seek to hit the baseball with great power. His concern, however, is not limited solely to the distance the ball travels, but also with the body music associated with the blow. The type he recognizes is the beautiful kinesthetic rhythm of his muscles contracting in precisely the proper sequence and the kinesthesia at the moment of contact.

With practice you can increase the pleasures of exercise by choosing a kinesthetic type that is rather difficult to achieve. When you do fulfill this goal, though, you'll be all the more thrilled for having done so. This is why the body music of a home run is so delightful to kinoartistically oriented people. They recognize they have achieved a difficult and uncommon kinesthetic type.

The idea that the pleasure associated with a type depends on its difficulty is not a modern one. In the auspicious year of 1776, for instance, James Boswell in his *Life of Johnson* wrote:

> *A man will hack half a year at a block of marble to make something in stone that hardly resembles a man. The value of statuary is owing to its difficulty. You would not value the finest head cut upon a carrot.*

Of course, as an artist, you should never expect to be successful at everything you try. But while failure is never particularly welcome, the degree of displeasure depends on the difficulty of a type. If you fail to fulfill a difficult type, you will experience little or no displeasure. This is why golfers do not get upset when they fail to make a hole-in-one.

On the other hand, failing a common or easily achieved type results in much displeasure. For verification all you have to do is watch a typical golfer who misses a six-inch putt.

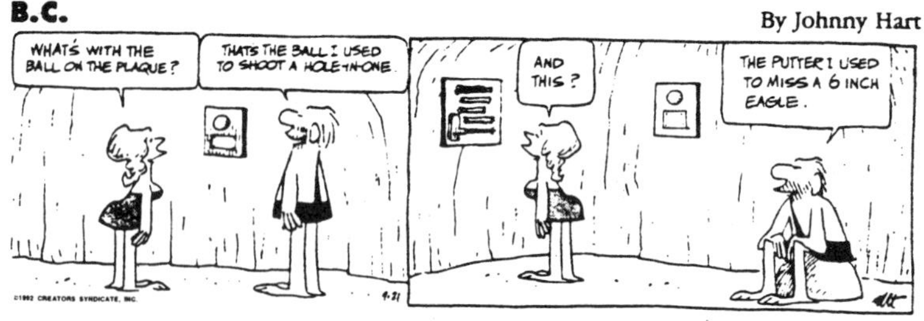

B.C. by permission of Johnny Hart and Creators Syndicate, Inc.

The use of the concepts discussed so far will help you successfully plan fulfilling and enjoyable exercise sessions. If you choose kinesthetic types—say, a one-finger hand stand—that are impossible to fulfill, your chances for receiving satisfaction are nil. Conversely, if types are too easily achieved (for example, tossing paper wads into a waste basket two feet away) there will be little satisfaction (i.e., boredom) in fulfilling them and much dissatisfaction should you fail. You are most likely to enjoy your body music if you choose types that are rather difficult but still within your capabilities. Naturally, as your kinoartistic abilities improve, you will want more difficult challenges.

Emotional Content

Even when a work of art has perfect technical form and is a magnificent type, it can still be vaguely unsatisfying. It can still lack something. That something is *emotional* content.

Though the intellectual content of art suggests a rational effort, the emotional content concerns the intuitive arousal of feelings. Just as it is difficult to imagine body music that has no meaning, it's hard to envision it as lacking emotion. Even in a simple exercise, say, an arm curl, you will at least have feelings of "like" or "dislike" toward its kinesthetic sensations.

To put emotional content into art, one needs vitality, will, and empathy. Kinoartists, especially, need a lot of vitality because no other artistic medium requires as much energy.

For the sake of efficiency, artists must control and give direction to their energy. As has already been stressed, kinoartists must be able to concentrate on their kinesthesia. The faculty of *will* is the emotional force behind this concentration. Will also allows people to persevere at an activity in spite of inevitable frustrations. Kinoartists will not always be satisfied with their art, but with practice their creations will continually improve. And remember that even a poor kinoartistic experience is far more satisfying than a physical activity with no esthetic appeal—as are most workouts.

Empathy is the ability of people to forget their own physical sensations and identify with those of another person or thing. An example is what happens when you watch someone suck on a juicy lemon—you can almost taste the lemon and your saliva starts flowing.

Another example of empathy occurs when a competing weight lifter strains under a heavy weight. Many audience members will hold their breath, tense their muscles, and clench their teeth right along with him. They are empathizing with his effort.

You are encouraged to try to empathize, kinesthetically, with other athletes. You might also try to empathize, kinesthetically, with animals and inanimate objects. Lifeless objects do not feel kinesthetic sensations, but that's okay. Because you have intelligence and feelings you will be able to create kinoartistic types by assuming that such objects do have kinesthesia.

The idea is not so far-fetched. In *Gardner's Art Through the Ages,* Horst de la Croix and Richard G. Tansey state:

> *In the prehistoric art of the caves, the rock paintings, and the art of Mesopotamia, we have admired the peculiar sensitivity of early artists to the animal. They seem to have empathized with the non-human animal, to have possessed . . . the power almost to share the being of the animals and to feel as it feels.*

Artists since then have also had the ability to empathize with their subjects. It is not unreasonable, therefore, to expect kinoartists to be able to create animal and non-animal types by imagining the subject's kinesthetic sensations. In other words, whereas painters can visualize nonhuman subjects such as animals or emotions, a kinoartist can kinolyze (another 'K' word) the same subjects. (Remember that word, kinolyze, and its meaning—imagining a subject's body music. It's vital to advanced kinoart.)

The James-Lange "Theory of Emotions" says an emotion is a group of sensations which have blended into a single quality—and this quality is perceived intuitively as a specific feeling.

For instance, when sky divers make their maiden jump they typically experience the sensations of non-support, off-balance, a rapid heart rate, involuntary breathholding, and a draining of blood from their face. Their mind automatically combines the sensations so that they are perceived as a single quality, which is intuitively interpretted as fear. They do not react logically and analytically toward the fused quality; they react emotionally—most likely with a sustained shriek.

To use the activity of "skipping" as an example of sensory fusion in kinoart, it's necessary to realize that practically every muscle is involved to either produce movement or stabilize a body part. Also, nearly every joint experiences some degree of movement. Each muscle contraction and joint movement produces a specific kinesthetic feeling. At every instant the kinesthesia, along with other sensations which arrive at the brain, are fused into a single quality that a person intuitively perceives as an emotion—probably joy. Incidentally, if you want to feel like a child again, try skipping. It will be a kinesthetic lollipop for you. The "Adult Rehabilitation Center" in the following cartoon could more accurately be called the "Kinesthetic Art Center."

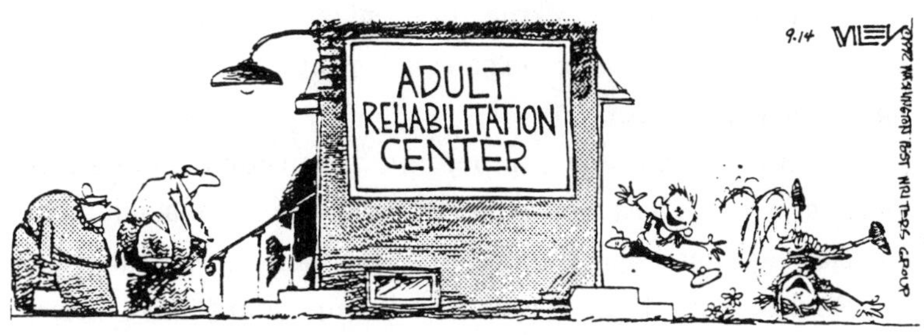

Initially, a person's emotional perception of jogging, or of any kinesthetic event, may be limited to simply pleasure or displeasure. However, the potential range of emotions that can be expressed and perceived in body music is as great as in any other artistic media. One of the major aims of kinoartists is to constantly increase the emotional content of their physical activity. Many ways for doing so appear later in this chapter and throughout the remainder of the book.

Jogging, admittedly, may not offer the range of emotional experiences that gymnastics or modern dance would. But jogging was chosen to show that even simple body music offers more than you might suspect. In one jogger, the total kinesthetic fusion may produce excitement or a sense of freedom. In another jogger, the same feelings along with sensations of labored breathing and a pounding heart may induce anxiety (especially if the jogger's younger brother or sister recently had a heart attack).

A person's body music will always have associated emotions, though they may at first be subliminal. Whether the emotions are positive or negative depends largely on the particular physical activity and one's perception of it. People can control their emotions by changing their perceptions, but a much easier and quicker way is to simply change the kinesthetic sensations to the brain. If jogging causes anxiety, a person can walk, play golf, shoot baskets, or take a leisurely swim.

A second, and extremely important, dimension of emotion is *moods.* Perhaps the best way to describe moods is to relate them to the sensations that cause moods. It is well known that different colors, sounds, sensations of touch, and temperatures have different effects on a person's mood. Prison cells painted "hot pink," for example, has a calming effect on inmates. The typeface of a book has an effect on the reader's emotions. The kinesthesia of different movements also tends to create different moods. A single strong muscle contraction will evoke one mood while a prolonged series of mild contractions will produce another.

The following table lists a number of movements and the moods they produce. (Of course, there is a vast number of variations between the extremes.) Remember, it is the kinesthesia associated with movements that actually affect moods, but it is easier to speak in terms of movements because they can be seen.

Movements for Producing Kinesthetic Feelings of Delicacy and Strength

Delicate	Strong
light resistance	heavy resistance
small movements	expansive movements
undulating movements	linear movements
grasping small objects	grasping large objects

Movements for Producing Kinesthetic Feelings of Calm and Excitement

Calm	Excitement
slow movements	quick movements
horizontal movements	diagonal/vertical movements
gentle curving movements	zig-zag movements
gentle gradation of movement	extreme contrasts in movements
symmetrically balanced patterns	unbalanced patterns
slow rhythms	rapid rhythms
subdued rhythms	staccato rhythms
even paced rhythms	irregularly paced rhythms

You can easily verify the previous lists by performing each of the movements and monitoring the effect on your mood. For a more powerful demonstration of the role of kinesthesia in creating moods, begin by whistling or singing the Christmas carol "Silent Night." You will find the lyrics and melody are calming. Then, accompany the song with the kinds of movements listed under "Excitement" in the previous table. It will be a confusing, disturbing esthetic experience because the moods produced by the song will conflict with those produced by the kinesthesia of your movements. To continue the experiment, you can accompany the song with the kinds of movements listed under "Calm." In this case, the moods produced by the song and the movement will be consistent and the harmony will generally be more esthetically satisfying.

You have considerable control over the emotional content of your body music because you can regulate the factors that affect emotions. With an intelligent choice of movements you can produce body music that creates specific sensory fusions and moods.

Emotions are also associated with your instinctive drives. And the strength of these emotions can be controlled by varying the intensity of the drives. It is quite common, for example, for people to crave activity after several days of inactivity—particularly if they are usually active. This is one reason why the joy of an activity tends to diminish if it's done day after day. To prevent this, you can engage in an activity every other day, or intersperse the activity with others—preferably with very different body music. More specifically, you can walk or jog on Mondays, Wednesdays, and Fridays and exercise with weights on Tuesdays and Saturdays. This is also an excellent fitness program.

A significant obstacle in dealing with the emotional content of art is the lack of a vocabulary that precisely describes feelings. The word "love," which can be used in a great many contexts, is a prime example of vocabulary inadequacy. You may love ice cream, love your dog, and love your significant other. But you would only want to marry one of these loves—presumably your significant other.

Kinoartists are doubly hampered. In addition to a limited emotional vocabulary, a kinesthetic vocabulary is practically nonexistent. Musicians, on the other hand, have exact names for musical notes. And painters have exact names for colors. That preciseness is a tremendous advantage in artistic communication. For one thing, it's very practical; it makes it a lot easier for an artist when ordering paint.

Kinesthetic artists do not completely lack a foundation for communication, however. They can rely on the science of kinesiology to help them get started in developing a language. Movements can occur at most of the joints in our bodies, though not in the same way in every joint. The three kinds of joint movements most people are aware of are flexion, extension, and rotation, but there are more than 20 other kinds—and many thousands of variations of these.

In addition to joints and movements, a kinoartistic language would have to take muscle tensions into consideration. Words such as weak, mild, moderate, strong, and intense are examples of terms that readily come to mind. The most difficult task in developing a body music language would be in selecting words for the various kinesthetic sensations.

Kinoart is a new artistic medium, though, and the kinesthetic terminology will undoubtedly become more extensive and accurate in due time. Until then, you will have to rely on the information in this book, common sense, intuition—and, frankly, a bit of faith to give you the confidence to control the emotional elements of your body music.

Components of Art Interrelate

The basic components of body music—design, pattern, and intellectual and emotional content—have been discussed separately. For organizational purposes this division is practical. It is not realistic, though, because every component of a work of art—form, meaning, and feeling—interrelates with the others.

Here's a simple example how meaning and emotion can be put into a physical event to create more captivating body music. First, stand flat-footed with your toes touching a line on the ground. Of course, the kinesthesia of this balanced event, though harmonious, will soon become boring. Lean forward from the ankles until you are just about to fall. The body music will be more interesting and the knowledge that you may lose your balance gives the sensations some meaning—namely, you could drive your nose three inches into the turf if you aren't careful. Even so, you realize all you have to do to regain your balance is step forward with one foot.

To add more meaning to the activity, stand at the edge of a swimming pool and again lean forward. Knowing you may fall into the water is certain to add some emotion. This very simple, but pleasant, kinoartistic experience of the calf muscles simultaneously stretching and contracting is guaranteed to produce plenty of meaning and emotion for you. An emotional climax occurs, of course, when you actually fall off-balance and plunge toward the water—especially if you're wearing your best clothes. (The event is also sure to arouse strong emotions in your companion, particularly if you're late for a first meeting with his or her parents.)

With just a little ingenuity, you can use esthetics to give practically every physical activity meaning and emotion. Specific exercise suggestions for helping you do this are given in Part Three. Exercise will be converted into satisfying and exciting kinoartistic sessions. You will quickly find that the body music approach to exercise certainly beats the dreaded 'W' word—working out.

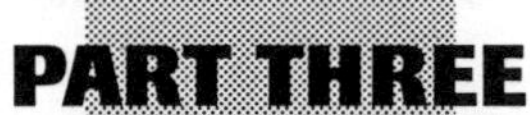

PART THREE

"Let each man exercise the art he knows."
Aristophanes

The body of knowledge presented in Part Two establishes the foundation for kinesthetic art. Briefly stated, you now know:

1. kinesthesia (kinesthetic sensations) does EXIST.
2. kinesthesia, or body music, has infinite VARIETY in terms of quality and quantity.
3. body music can be CONTROLLED because the joint movements and muscular tensions that produce body music can be controlled.
4. ART can be defined as something that is perceived through the senses, is organized toward a unified experience, and has esthetic appeal.
5. body music can be PERCEIVED.
6. kinesthesia can be arranged into UNIFIED PATTERNS.
7. unified kinesthetic patterns can have ESTHETIC APPEAL.
8. kinesthetic patterns can be consciously associated with types to give the patterns INTELLECTUAL CONTENT.
9. kinesthetic patterns can intuitively arouse EMOTIONAL FEELINGS.

10. when perceived kinesthetic sensations are organized into a unified experience with esthetic appeal the result is kinesthetic art (KINOART) or body music.

With these foundations, you can proceed with confidence in converting your workouts to gratifying body music compositions. Although much information has been presented to help you do this (perhaps more than you think you will ever need), the basic information is actually only a small fraction of what could have been offered. You will probably find yourself often turning back to the previous chapters for helpful ideas to improve your body music. The purpose of Part Three is to give many more specific suggestions on how you can apply the information to a wide range of physical activities.

Even though these suggestions are based on esthetics, they are still only suggestions. Great artists go beyond established guidelines and broaden the concepts of art. However, these masters invariably begin their careers by studying and following the standards of their time. Picasso is a classic example. His earliest paintings were quite realistic. Then he went through an impressionistic phase, which was popular at the time. After finding even that style confining and unfulfilling, he blazed his own trail, which led to cubism.

You are strongly advised to take a similar route. That is, start by following the principles of esthetics as they are presented in this book. Then, as you gain experience you can deviate from the guidelines *if* they hinder your creativity and self-expression.

A word of reserve is offered. Namely, no one embarking on an artistic quest should expect miracles. A beginning violinist will not be able to play as well as Jascha Heifetz. A novice would do well to play a single pure note. But with diligent practice, one can cultivate innate abilities. Practice is the key.

Painters have to practice mixing paint for the color sensations they want. Then they have to organize them into esthetic configurations to produce a work of art. As a kinoartist, you have similar aims. You have to practice creating and organizing kinesthetic sensations (the body's music) into esthetic patterns. Your instrument, of course, is your body and your "keyboard" consists of joints movements and muscular tensions. As mentioned earlier, though, your instrument is not limited to 88 keys. It has more than 600 "keys" when counting just the muscles—not taking the 200 joints into consideration.

Admittedly, it is not easy to become an accomplished painter, musician, or kinoartist. Besides the concentration required, there may be periods of frustration. Further, depending on one's talents and motivations, some people will have greater success than others. Everyone, however, can improve and achieve some artistic fulfillment in any medium.

Body music is as different from "working out" as painting a picture is from painting a barn. Yet, the activities in a body music session can be exactly the same as those in a traditional workout. The difference is in a person's goals and attitude. In a workout, improved health, fitness, and appearance are typically sought. In kinoart, activities are planned according to esthetics with the goal being an artistic kinesthetic experience. Ironically, though, the traditional goals of exercise will be achieved more easily with the body music approach because the creative exercise sessions will be far more satisfying and enjoyable.

Because it is not within the scope of this book to apply kinoart to every single sport and exercise, seven categories have been formed. Virtually every type of exercise will fall within one of them. Although a separate chapter has been devoted to each category, many of the suggestions can be applied from one category to another.

This book does not explain how to lift weights, jog, play tennis, dance, or whatever. It is presumed you are fairly knowledgeable and skillful in your chosen activity. The aim of this book is to show how you can change your approach and attitude toward an activity so it becomes a satisfying kinoartistic experience—in addition to achieving its traditional benefits.

EXPLORATORY EXERCISES

7

Before converting your workouts to kinoart, it pays to do some exploratory activities to get more in touch with your body music. I've found that people find much enjoyment even in this initial stage of kinoart.

A good way to begin is with the luxuriously exaggerated yawn mentioned previously. It is a delicious kinesthetic event that anyone can appreciate. Closing your eyes during this or any activity helps you experience the body music more keenly because it eliminates extraneous sensations that might mask subtle kinesthetic sensations.

After yawning, you can move to a mat or bed—but not to sleep. Start by lying on your back with a pillow under your knees. Then contract one muscle group at a time while stretching the opposing muscle group. For instance, if you extend your leg forward by contracting the muscles on the front of the thigh, the muscles on the back of the thigh will be stretching.

At the same time *concentrate* on the kinesthesia associated with the contractions and stretches. It's easier to keep track of your progress if you begin at your toes and proceed toward your head. After gently curling the toes of your right foot, relax them briefly and curl them with moderate force. Relax again and then curl them with even more force. The kinesthetic differences in the gradation design of this pattern will be striking. Then do the same exercise with your left foot. Or you could alternate single contractions between your left and right side. Next, create a similar elementary pattern by pointing your right foot. You'll feel your calf muscles contracting. After you have worked your way up to the muscles of your jaw and face, try contracting the muscles of both feet simultaneously and again work your way up from the toes to the head.

With exercises such as these, you introduce yourself to your kinesthetic keyboard. In addition, you create a kinesthetic work of art consisting of a gradation design that repeats itself to form similar elementary patterns. You can create more complex body music by combining contractions of muscles in different parts of the body. These kinoart examples may sound simple, but paintings with far less esthetic substance have won awards. For example, for a 1993 New York City exhibition, an artist presented a totally white canvas. An ecstatic art critic said the artist was the ultimate "minimalist." Well, if that's true, I suppose a person lying on a bed could be called a kinoartistic minimalist.

In exploratory sessions, strive to expand the awareness of your kinesthesia. Such exercises should prove to be very enlightening. The body's joints are capable of extraordinary movements by varying direction, speed, range, and quality (e.g., fast or slow). Your muscles, due to variations in both contractions *and* stretches, are capable of an equally wide range of tensions. The combinations of movements and tensions are infinite—and each combination feels kinesthetically unique.

A specific illustration of how to further explore your body music is shown in Fig. 7-1. Begin by lying on your back. First, bring your legs to position (B). Then extend them to (C). Next, lower them to (D). Return to (C) and lower your legs laterally (E). Stretch the muscles, but not to the point of discomfort. After returning your legs once again to (C), rock them from side to side (F) or move them in a circular fashion (G).

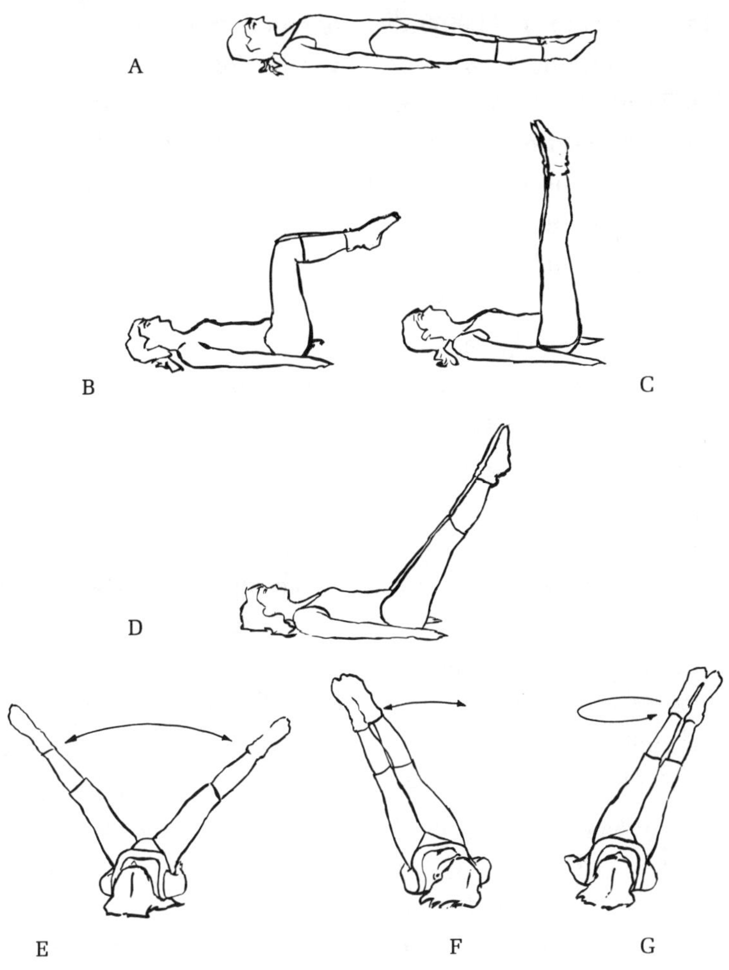

Fig. 7-1. Getting Acquainted with Your Kinesthesia.

There are many possible variations of these leg exercises. The precise ones are not important as long as you concentrate on the body music. Esthetically, it's best to initially limit the repetitions of each movement to one or two. As your kinesthetic attention improves, you may find four or five repetitions more appealing or perhaps even as many as seven or eight. This is not a competition, however—eight is not better than four, or even one.

Corresponding movements may be performed with the arms alone. Then more complex kinesthetic patterns may be created by *superimposing* arm movements on those of the legs and trunk.

To superimpose a variety of balance patterns, movements can be performed, first, while standing firmly on both feet. Then the same exercises can be done with one foot on a bench. To further increase the kinesthetic interest, movements can be done with the eyes closed. The heightened effect is amazing.

You may be surprised to find that exploratory movements can be subtle, almost visually imperceptible, and still be very meaningful and emotionally powerful. This is particularly true if the muscular contractions or stretches are very intense. For a demonstration, sit down and put your palms together a few inches in front of your chest; let your forearms hang at an angle of about 45°. Then push your palms together while slowly raising your elbows upward and downward (a few inches) in a flapping motion. Close your eyes and *concentrate* on your body music. I can't know exactly what you'll feel, but you should feel something. The first time I did this I was astounded to feel as if I were actually flying. It wasn't long before a pterodactyl came to mind. It was a wonderful experience I can duplicate anytime.

No, I hadn't been imbibing. And I'm not mystic, by any means. In fact, my daughters, with ill-disguised disgust, sometimes accuse me of being a very conservative fellow. (Actually, "square" is the term they use, and they're probably right.) But I do have an imagination. I'm sure the pterodactyl popped into my mind because I had just read *Jurassic Park* by Michael Crichton. That is an example of art inspiring art, a technique you may find useful.

Later, I experimented by positioning my palms in front of my neck instead of my chest. A sparrow hawk entered my mind, not visually but kinesthetically. I *concentrated* on feeling what I thought a sparrow hawk would feel if it concentrated on its kinesthesia. In other words, I was not visualizing—I was kinolyzing. If this sounds weird to you, rest assured that it seemed a tad strange to me, too, at first. But kinolyzing creates an incredibly delightful experience—making exercising far more enjoyable than it normally is. My students seem to enjoy kinolyzing more than any other aspect of kinoart (perhaps because it requires imagination and creativity).

These exploratory activities are merely suggestions for helping you to get closer to your body music. You are strongly encouraged to experiment and create your own kinoartistic designs and patterns. A review of Chapters Five and Six (Form and Content) will be very helpful.

CALISTHENICS

8

The word "calisthenics" comes from two ancient Greek words—*kallos*, meaning beauty, and *sthenos*, meaning strength. Indeed, most dictionaries define calisthenics as exercises that develop a strong and graceful body—without the use of equipment.

Even though calisthenics have these traditional aims, they can at the same time result in body music. All you have to do is use the laws of esthetics in planning the exercises. There is absolutely no conflict. The guidelines will enhance calisthenics by making them kinesthetically more interesting.

Suggestions for applying esthetics to calisthenics are shown in this chapter for a few specific exercises. With some imagination the advice can be used for all other calisthenic exercises.

Fig. 8-1 shows the starting position for a basic shoulder exercise. Keeping your wrists rigid, bring your arms forward so your fingers touch or nearly touch at (B). Then return your arms to (A). The tension in your shoulder muscles will vary and create a gradation design from one repetition to another. As always, *concentrate* on your body music. At first, repeat this action slowly—two times. When you feel you can successfully concentrate on more repetitions, the number can gradually be increased—to a maximum of eight, if you wish.

The number of repetitions is up to you. I've found that three is a number I can easily handle. Five repetitions is difficult. For some reason I rarely think of doing four. Maybe that's because odd numbers are thought to be more artistic than even ones. At any rate, the number of repetitions should never be for competition. There's no magic number. If you perform two repetitions and can successfully concentrate on their kinesthetic sensations and really feel them, you are far better off than a person who does eight repetitions but has difficulty focusing on the sensations.

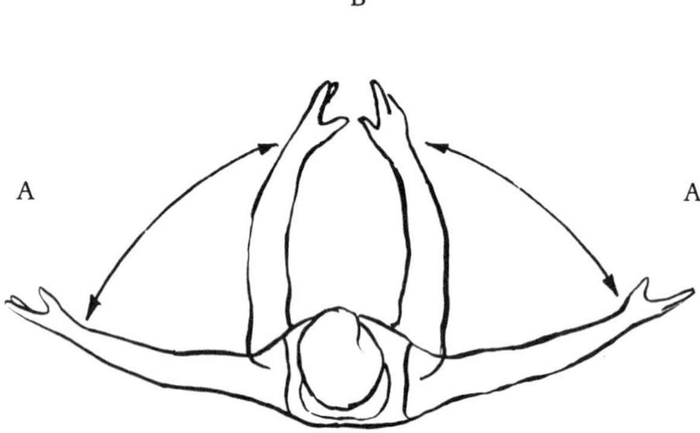

Fig. 8-1. A Basic Shoulder Exercise with Rigid Wrists (overhead view).

To increase the esthetic appeal of the basic shoulder exercise, do the movements with more flexible elbow and wrist actions. The illustration in Fig. 8-2 shows how the elbows and wrists can lead the way with the hands and fingers lagging behind. Later, you can superimpose exaggerated thrusting of the chest forward and backward (or any direction) for some wonderful kinesthesia. In both cases, the complex and rhythmic patterns of your body music will be surprisingly different and far more exciting than those of the basic shoulder exercise alone.

True, some men may feel these movements are too dance-like. Well, if a man feels that insecure about his masculinity, maybe he had best limit his activity to watching football. But the fact is, dancing has both masculine and feminine roles. That applies to social dancing and ballet. I don't suggest that men strap on toe shoes and perform *fouettés*. But graceful movements do not need to be effeminate—just watch the top football, basketball, and baseball players in action. There are moments when they are as graceful as ballet dancers.

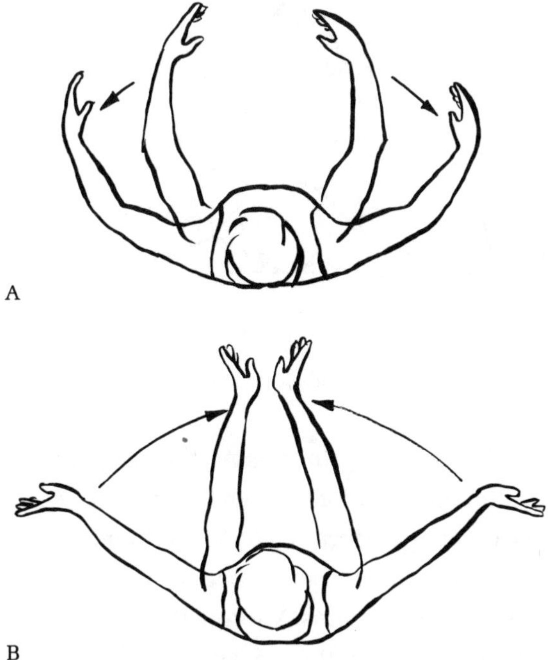

Fig. 8-2. A Shoulder Exercise with Flexible Wrists.

Many variations in design are possible with these basic shoulder exercises. The degree of kinesthetic contrast can be increased by alternating the expansive motions of (B), in Fig. 8-3, with the reduced range of the movement shown in (A).

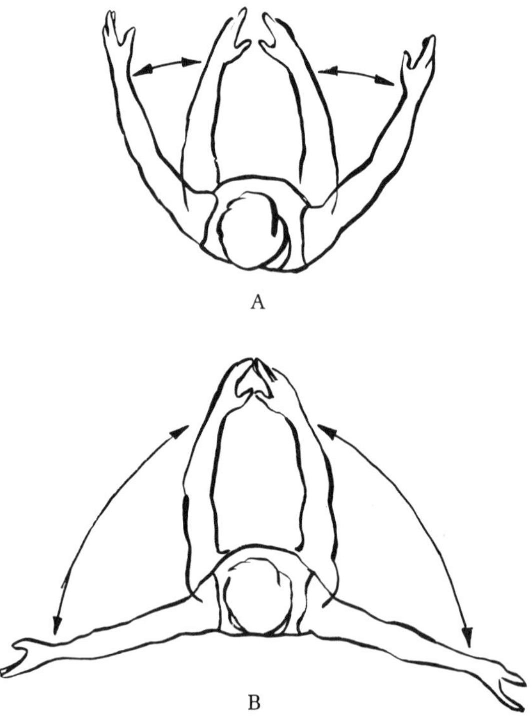

Fig. 8-3. Reduced Movements (A) and Expansive Movements (B).

Moreover, by gradually increasing the range of movement, another kinesthetic gradation design is created. An extended pattern can be done by performing one repetition, then a group of two, then a group of three, and so on, with brief periods of restraint (relaxation) between the groups. Varying the speed of motion can produce a rhythmic effect that makes the exercise still more inviting.

Several variations-on-a-theme for shoulder exercises are shown in Fig. 8-4 on the next page. You can extend your arms horizontally to the sides (A) and alternately raise and lower them, either in unison for a symmetrically balanced pattern or out-of-phase for an asymmetrically balanced pattern. The arms and wrists can be rigid or they can be flexible to resemble the flapping motions of a bird's wings. Similar motions can be done with your arms extended overhead (B) or horizontally to the front (C) or from a bent-over stance (D).

Gradations can be combined by progressing from one basic pattern to another. An attractive kinesthetic pattern is produced when you rotate your arms in a circular path in any one of the variations. The arms may circle in the same direction as depicted in (E) or in opposite directions.

In addition, the size of the circles can be changed rapidly or gradually. By controlling the movements, you control your body music. If the sensations are not satisfying, merely experiment until they are—using the laws of esthetics to ensure a sense of harmony.

You can see that with kinoart, exercise is not merely a rigid physical experience. The approach involves the brain and the soul. Once you "get into it," you'll discover body music can set you free.

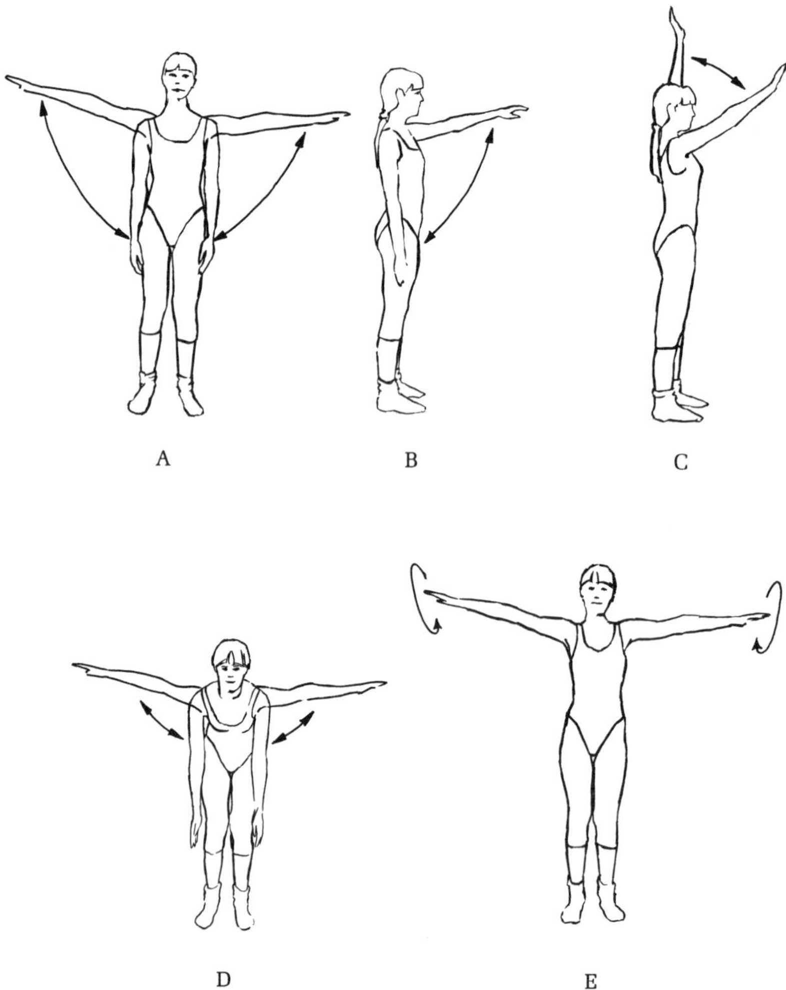

Fig. 8-4. Variations-on-a-Theme for Shoulder Exercises.

Some form variations that are not easily created with shoulder exercises are shown in Fig. 8-5 with leg (quadriceps) exercises. The body music of a basic knee bend can be changed by varying the degree of knee-bend. If you're strong enough, one leg knee bends (B) can also be done—using a chair under your rear end for safety.

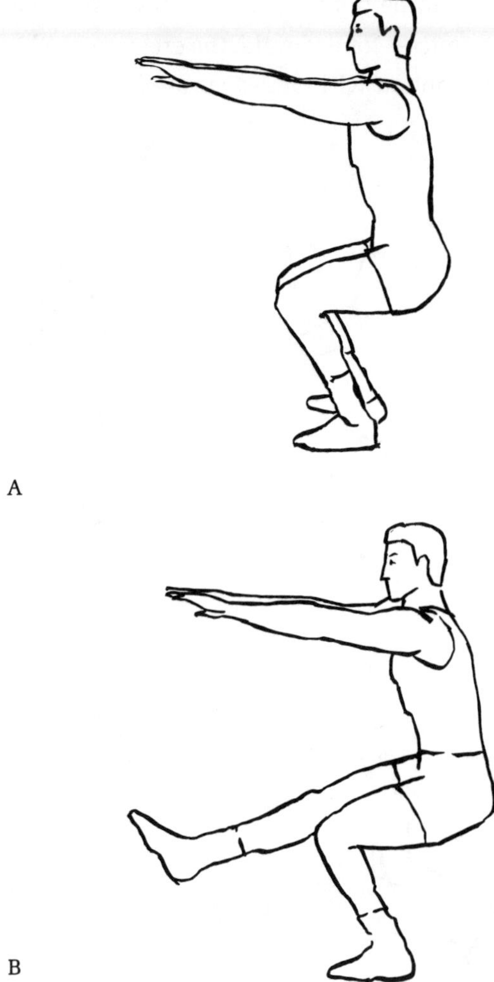

Fig. 8-5. Basic Knee Bend.

Other variations include leaning forward or backward a bit while doing a knee bend. A combination of the two (Fig. 8-6) creates an especially provocative kinesthetic pattern. That is, lean forward on the way down, and on the way up lean back and thrust your hips forward. Arm and head motions may be added and the entire movement can be done to add intellectual content to the kinesthetic experience—for example, the creation of a kinesthetic cobra. Emotional content will almost surely follow.

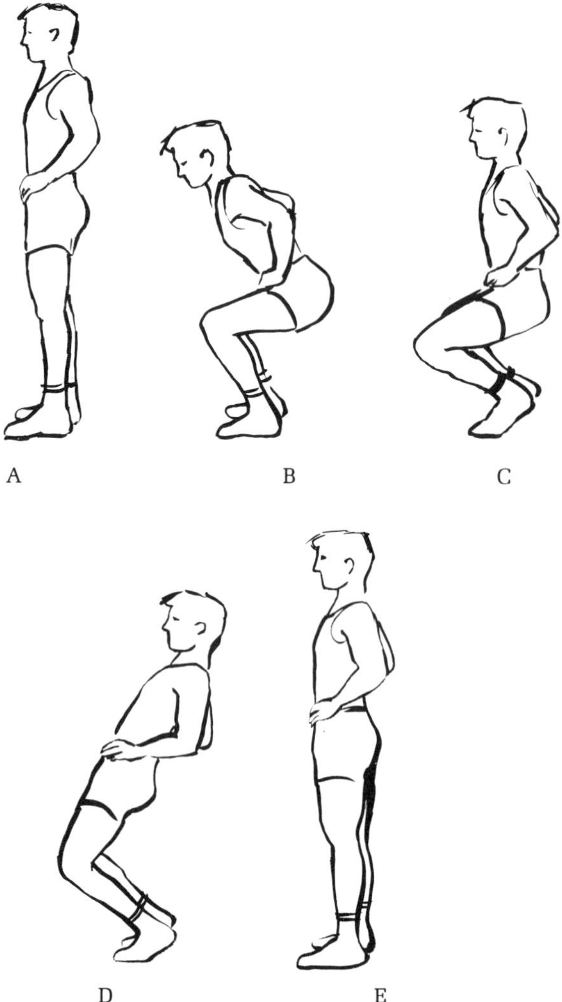

Fig. 8-6. Forward and Backward Knee Bend Combination (symmetrically balanced).

Interesting body music can be created when you rock from side to side (Fig. 8-7) so your weight is primarily on one foot as in (B), and then the other (D). An even more complex and fascinating body music composition is made when the knee-bend patterns in Fig. 8-6 and Fig. 8-7 are superimposed on one another.

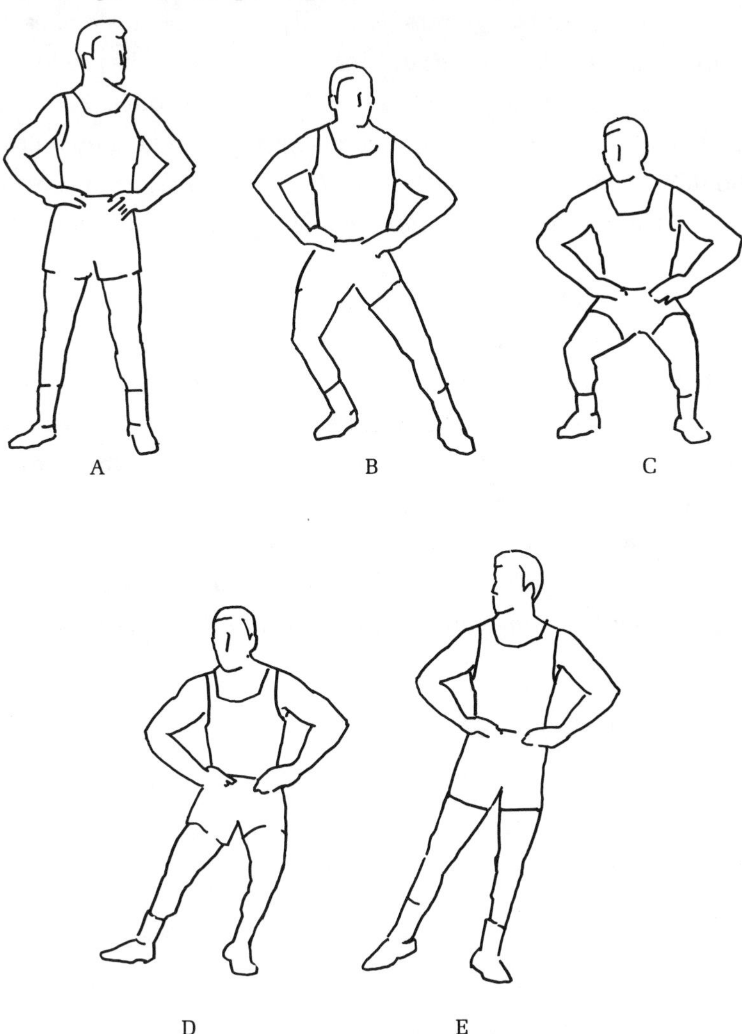

Fig. 8-7. Side-to-Side Knee Bend Variation (asymmetrically balanced).

Knee bends, like all exercises, can vary greatly in terms of speed and force. If the leg muscles contract forcefully and quickly enough, the result will be a jump. Three kinds of jumps are shown in Fig. 8-8. In (A) the woman keeps her feet close together; in (B) she alternates them in a forward and back position; and in (C) she keeps them spread apart to the sides. Naturally, the body music of each type of jump is different and additional variations can be produced by forming combination patterns with them and other kinds of movements. For example, superimposing any kind of jump onto a shoulder exercise similar to that shown in Fig. 8-4(A) would create a kind of jumping jack or an imitation of a gooney bird attempting to take off. The chief difference between a regular calisthenics jumping jack and a kinoartistic jumping jack is kinesthetic concentration—but, oh, the difference in pleasure!

Differences in the balance patterns of all knee bend exercises can be produced by either doing them flat-footed or on the balls of the feet. Another way is to lean forward, backward, or to the sides—practically off-balance.

Most calisthenic exercises can be done in the water. The body music, however, will be much different because the water offers more resistance to movement than air, and a greater range of muscle tension is possible.

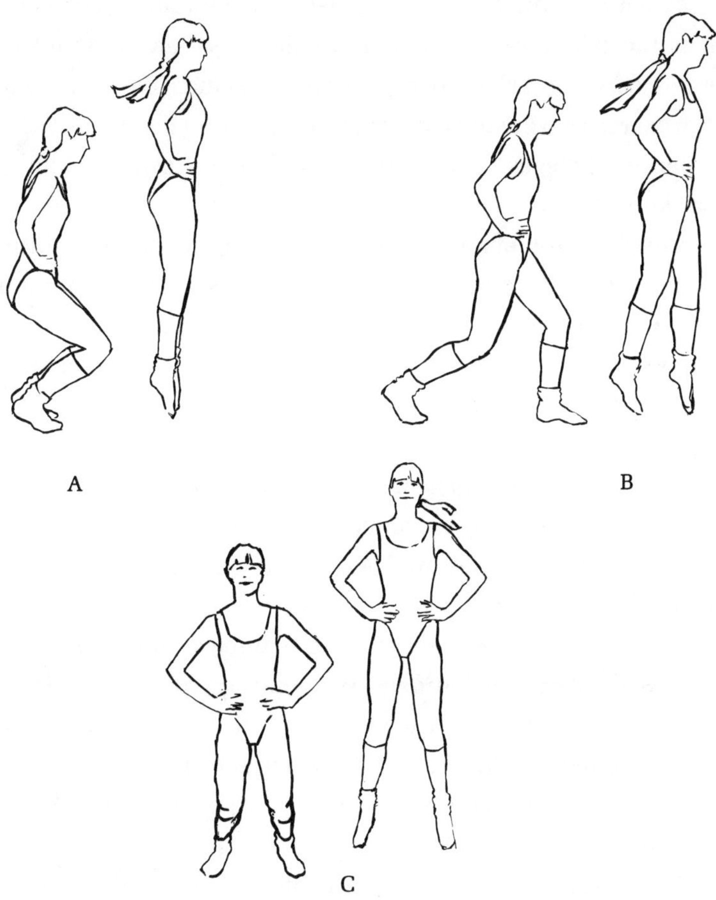

Fig. 8-8. Three Kinds of Jumps.

Traditional calisthenic programs tend to lose their allure rather quickly. Many people have complained to me that they just can't stick with a traditional calisthenics program. But the kinesthetic methods presented here will counteract the boredom.

Aerobic dance programs, which are essentially calisthenics, are also designed to reduce boredom. Most people believe it is the music that makes aerobic classes palatable. However, another reason aerobic dance is more enjoyable than traditional calisthenics is the wider variety of kinesthetic sensations produced by aerobic dancing. The body music would be much clearer, though, if the exercises were not performed so fast. Slowing down, at least in the initial stages, would allow people to concentrate more on their kinesthesia.

Another problem with aerobic dancing is the ear-splitting volume of the music and the leader's voice commands that usually completely mask the dancers' kinesthetic sensations. Fortunately, these negative aspects can easily be reduced or eliminated. Ear plugs work nicely.

Aerobic dancing can be a fine kinoartistic activity. Its only artistic drawback is that one person choreographs the same routine for everyone. The leader can be compared to an artist who creates "paint-by-the-number" canvases. And aerobic students are the people who "paint" the numbered spaces. Although the students may be having fun (which is desirable), the aerobic "puppets" surely cannot be considered artistic. If the dancers would approach their aerobic sessions as kinoartists, they would have even more fun, because the creative aspects would greatly add to their satisfaction.

Of course, the adaptation of kinoart to aerobics would require more individualized guidance by aerobic leaders. Each dancer would be encouraged to choreograph his or her own routine, which would be based on individual interests and capabilities. Even in large classes there is no reason why individuals cannot move on their own and develop kinoartistic routines with intellectual and emotional content. It would simply require more organizational skill and effort by the class leader and, of course, an understanding of body music.

REPETITIOUS EXERCISES

9

Walking, jogging, rope jumping, stairwalking, bicycling, cross-country skiing, swimming, rowing, and skating are all examples of activities consisting of prolonged series of repetitions. Because there's little variety in these events, the associated body music is monotonous. Most people, therefore, think the activities are boring.

This same kinesthetic monotony, however, can be quite appealing. People whose lives are in constant turmoil usually find considerable relief in the orderliness (the calming effect) of repetition. Examples might be a harried parent with a herd of rambunctious offspring or a business person struggling with mountains of paperwork, bureaucratic absurdities, and jangling telephones. If these people, while walking or jogging, would concentrate on the orderly, repetitious flow of their body music, they would magnify the soothing effect of the activities. Kinolyzing objects such as clocks or metronomes would help even further. Similar to visualizing, kinolyzing is done by imagining an object's kinesthetic sensations and then attempting to duplicate them with your own.

Don't worry about failure in kinolyzing. First of all, no one will ever know how successful you are. Secondly, even if you are only slightly successful, it can make exercise more enjoyable. And finally, practice leads to the improved ability to kinolyze.

As indicated earlier, most people who are attracted to the fitness benefits of repetitive activities would prefer the events to be more exciting. Need proof? Just watch a group of children walking. Typically, their normal walking steps are liberally interspersed with walking backward and sideways, skipping, leaping, jumping, balancing along a curb or railroad track, jogging, sprinting, and galloping. They may even swing both arms forward and back at the same time, or swing each arm forward and back along with the leg on the same side. Walking is clearly not boring to them. It is an adventure. This is possible because children typically are not inhibited about the way they move.

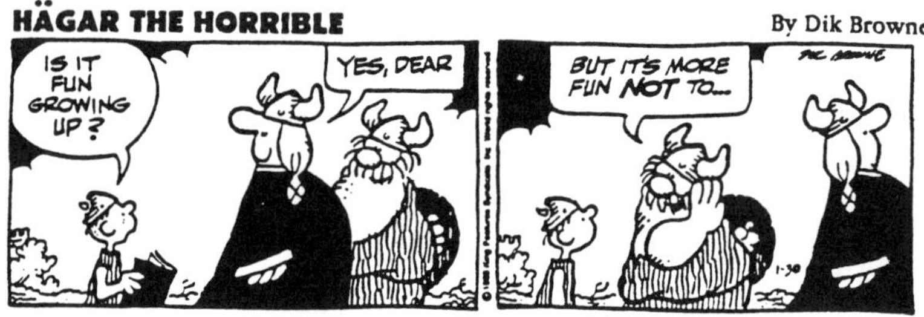

HAGAR—Reprinted by permission. King Features Syndicate, Inc.

As J.E. Springard wrote in *Creative Criticism,* letting oneself go is what art is always aiming at. Youngsters embrace this idea by intuitively transforming their walks into kinoart without realizing it. They do not know they are creating body music; they just know walking feels good—and using a variety of steps is downright fun and exciting.

In a prolonged series of steps, it doesn't take much variation (in either number or quality) to create a vastly more interesting kinesthetic effect. This can be easily demonstrated by using a visual example. The series of identical gray circles (Fig. 9-1) are comparable to a series of identical footsteps.

Now, compare the series of identical circles with Chuck Close's *Self-Portrait* (Fig. 9-2). The artist merely varied the shadings of the circles. Interestingly, not only do the variations make the painting more interesting, a visual *type* is created—a face—and the pattern is filled with intellectual content. The emotional content (how one feels about the painting) will vary according to the viewer. For instance, some people may like the painting, others may dislike it. Some may think the face has a benign quality, others may think it has a sinister one, etc.

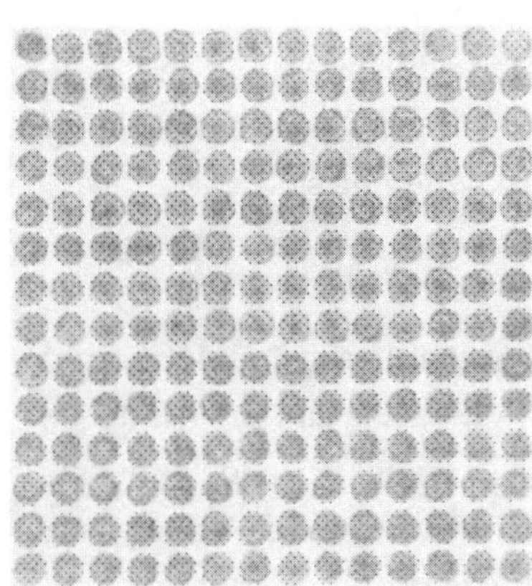

Fig. 9-1. Series of Identical Circles.

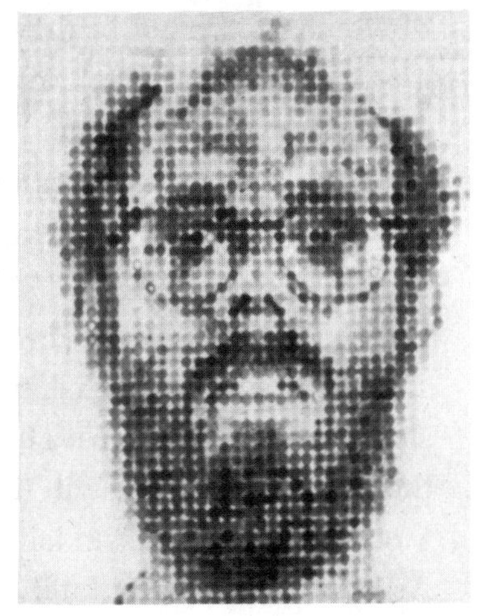

Fig. 9-2. Chuck Close. *Self-Portrait.* 1991. Memphis Brooks Museum of Art.

Merely by varying a repetitious pattern, Chuck Close created an effect that is so engaging it is almost mesmerizing. In much the same way, you can create fascinating body music by putting variations in a repetitious activity such as walking. Again, it helps immeasurably if you concentrate on the sensations.

If childhood walking experiences are so delightful, why doesn't the attitude carry over into adulthood? Insight may be gained by observing a child walking with a parent. Handholding may at times be an important safety measure, but it certainly stifles a child's natural desire for a variety of movement experiences. Commands such as, "Stop that silly galloping!" "Get off the curb, you're not a goat!" and "You're going to hurt yourself!" do not help either.

Part of the problem may be that children are too intelligent. They learn well, so they are easily molded. By their teens, they are well on their way to having internalized society's rules, the chief of which is, "Do not be different!"

Society tends to look down on those who dare to be themselves. Maybe society is frightened by a person who dares to be independent. At any rate, pressures comes from all sides to conform. Henry David Thoreau, however, hit the mark when he said:

> *Let him keep step to the music which he hears, however measured or far away.*

The adage has long been popular, but adhering to it is another story. People with great strength of character can choose to be themselves—but they will usually pay a social price for doing so. Most people understandably are not willing to pay the price. Artists, however, absolutely must. It is part of their artistic dues.

Children who grow up and manage to retain their ability to play freely become artists. As McCarter and Gilbert say in *Living with Art:*

> *"We might speculate that there is something of the child in all artists. Not in the sense of immaturity or lack of intellectual development, but in the ability to experiment uncensored by conventional standards of good and bad. . . . Could it be that the artist lives in all of us until and unless something destroys it?"*

That last sentence, if true, is enough to make me cry. In an optimistic vein, though, let's assume that the freedom to express oneself cannot be totally destroyed—only driven underground. Even in adulthood, therefore, it's not too late to make walking more interesting and artistic. It does require "letting go," though, and some people may be embarrassed by how they look. The idea is to begin with more subtle kinesthetic variations.

When the local swimming pool is closed, I'll walk around the track for a few miles. I also walk to and from work. Wherever, I use a lot of variations to make the body music associated with walking more interesting. Sometimes I carry a horseshoe, which I swing forward and back and pass it (or toss it) from one hand to another. Besides being a nice kinoartistic event, it's an excellent exercise.

If it's raining, I'll walk around an indoor basketball court. Many times I'll spontaneously use at least 50 or 60 walking variations in a half hour. With a radio blaring rock music in the background, it's not that difficult to create new ways of moving.

Often I will racewalk (also called striding). That's where you swivel your hips in an exaggerated fashion and pump your bent arms. True, you may look like a rooster on his way to a "hot" date. But striding is far more interesting, kinesthetically, than regular walking. You can vary the sensations considerably with such motions by leaning a bit forward at the waist, by standing very erect, or even by arching backward a bit.

If there are people around and I'm in a shy mood (it happens), I'll use a modified version. I swivel my hips just a bit more than usual, and when my arms swing to the rear, I extend them rather forcefully. It doesn't take long for the triceps to wake up and start "singing." The combination of hip rotation and triceps extension feels a bit awkward at first, but soon smooths out.

On these movements I superimpose a side-to-side leaning motion at the waist. Once mastered, this merger of motions is really absorbing and fun. This is just one variation, hundreds of others can be created with a little imagination. And bear in mind that walkers are very tolerant and stick together. Perhaps it's because some of their sedentary friends think walkers in general are a "few inches short of a full stride." Still, there are 67.8 million walkers, making it the number one fitness activity, according to the National Sporting Goods Association.

Jogging, like walking, can be more esthetically stimulating by adding variety. That variety is one reason why cross-country jogging is more appealing than jogging on a track. The body music associated with running at varying speeds, up and down hills, and on surfaces with different textures and "give" adds interest.

Even track running can be made far more interesting by applying the same variations as for walking, which certainly will not detract from the cardiovascular benefits joggers seek. Some simple variations include moving backward, sideways, leaning from side to side, and accentuating every third or fifth step.

Walking or jogging in a pool with water up to the chest, or even the chin, greatly changes the body music of the activity because your weight is reduced to a few pounds. It's easy to kinolyze that you are walking or jogging on the moon—into a stiff head wind (assuming the moon had an atmosphere). You won't be able to walk or run very rapidly in the pool, but who cares? It's the exercise and its kinesthesia you are concerned with. You can, of course, perform a variety of movements with the arms as well as the legs. Many swimming centers are now providing water aerobics classes. Besides being an excellent low-injury exercise, this fairly new activity offers a rich potential for body music compositions.

Kinesthetic diversity can also be produced while bicycling by speeding up and slowing down, going up and down hills, turning corners, and riding over different surfaces. If you want structured kinesthetic patterns, use the ideas of design and form. One suggestion is to pedal with increased force on every third (or fifth) half-cycle so the forceful element alternates from side to side. You can also rock your body forward at the waist and swing your elbows forward with each cycle or every third (or fifth) cycle of the pedals. Head movements, too, can be superimposed to enrich the body music of cycling. Variations include bobbing forward and back, side to side, and circular motions.

The kinesthetic aura of balance can be rhythmically varied by swerving from side to side on a regular bicycle. You can pedal, or coast with your feet on the pedals, or extend your legs laterally.

It is not difficult to associate the kinesthesia of bicycling with that of a swooping bird, a galloping horse, a race car, or some other rapidly moving type. Such kinolyzing puts intellectual content in kinoart. Emotional content ranging from an exhilarating sense of freedom to a fear of falling off-balance will often appear in the kinoart of cycling without you even trying.

You do not always have to put intellectual and emotional content in your kinoart. While those are the ultimate esthetic adventures, kinoart based completely on form (design and pattern) can also be quite pleasant. In any event, you must always concentrate on your kinesthesia (body music).

Okay, not always. *Safety* is a higher priority than art. If you are bicycling on a busy street, do not even think about esthetics. Pretend you're in a jungle full of crazed beasts—not a bad analogy if you think about it—and devote your full attention to survival.

Some artists find it difficult to concentrate on their work when people are watching. Kinoartists are no exception. In this regard rope jumpers have an advantage over walkers, joggers, and bicyclists. They can practice in the privacy of their homes.

The following illustrations (Fig. 9-3) show just a few of the rope jumping patterns that can be combined with the basic forward jumping pattern. The variations can also be used to create design gradations based upon complexity. The kinesthetic sensations, of course, will vary greatly with different movement patterns.

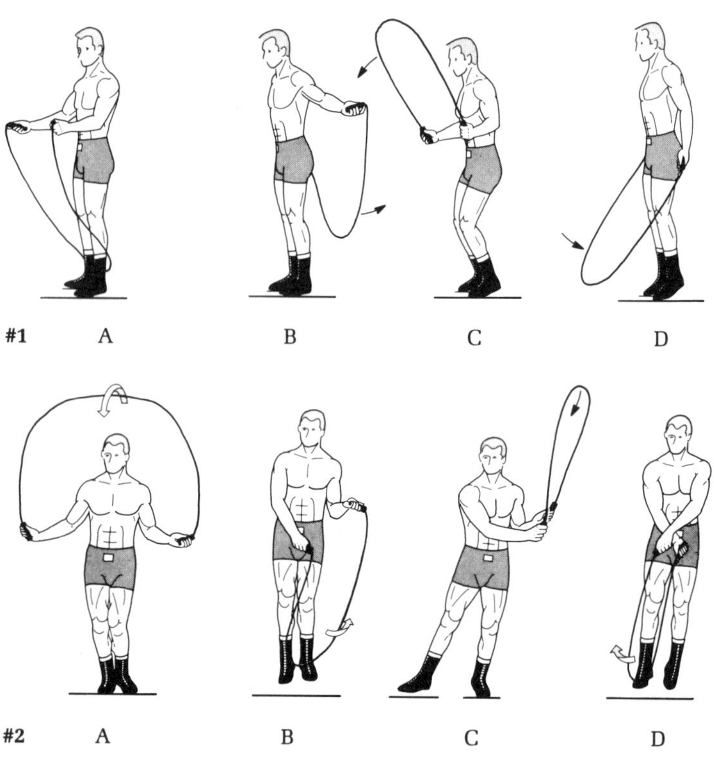

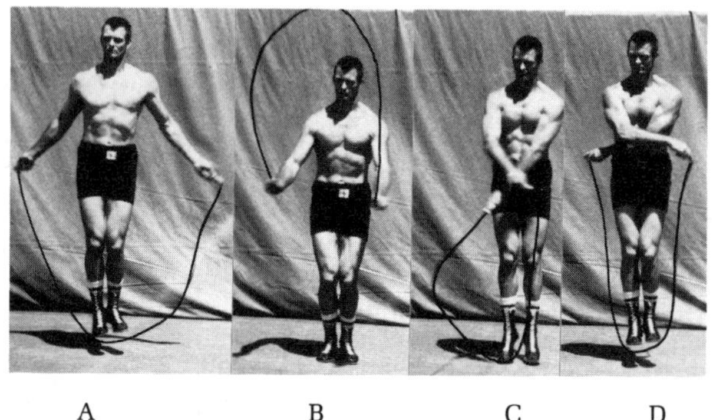

Fig. 9-3. Three Rope Jumping Variations.

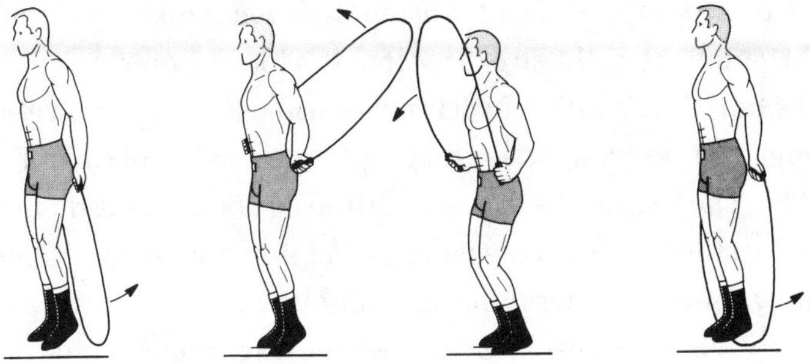

E F G H

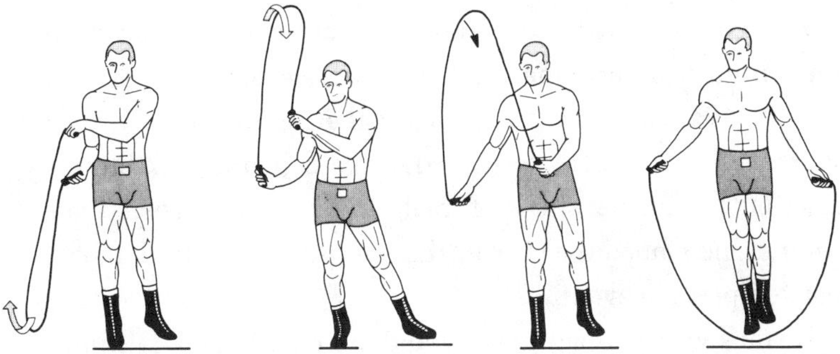

E F G H

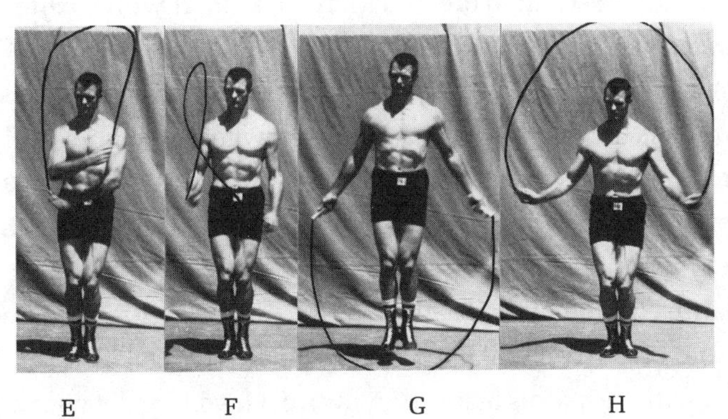

E F G H

Swimmers can expand the diversity of their body music and make it more stimulating by using different strokes and making slight variations to the strokes. Already a lot of people do this "just for the fun of it." That's why it is not unusual to see a person gliding through the water with alternating front crawl strokes and back strokes. The reason it's fun is that it feels good—kinesthetically. The kinesthetic attractiveness of swimming can be multiplied by creating complex patterns that include alternating strokes of breast, butterfly, side, and back strokes. Easier ways include alternating breathing from one side to the other and alternating fast laps, or strokes, with slow ones.

Anyone can create unusual body music compositions merely by inventing new movements. Some years ago one of my graduate students, Walter Casey, did exactly that as his project in my biomechanics class. His stroke could be called a back butterfly stroke, but in a further stroke of creativity, and with his usual sense of humor, he named the stroke "the mosquito." It would make an great competitive event.

If you swim competitively, you don't have a lot of latitude as far as movements are concerned. Your coach will see to that. But if you're a recreational swimmer, you can swim any way you want. You have the freedom to create satisfying kinoart while achieving the fitness benefits you want.

An excellent way to expand the kinesthetic sensations of swimming is to wear swim fins. They allow for more powerful leg and ankle "music." A very simple contrast pattern can be created by alternating laps where you only use your arms with laps where you only use your legs.

Mainly, though, fins free the hands to do untraditional maneuvers—and create original body music. Your arms can be extended forward with the palms facing downward. Or you can let your arms drag behind, or extend them to the side like airplane wings. With arms at a 45° angle you're a jet with swept-back wings. In all these cases, interesting kinesthetic and skin sensations can be achieved with waving or fluttering motions of the hands.

The burning question that emerges from this discussion is, "Can the body music associated with these repetitious activities really be considered artistic?" The simple answer is, "Of course." Prolonged series of repetitions are often seen in traditional art. Andy Warhol's wall-sized *210 Coca-Cola Bottles* immediately comes to mind. As the name suggests, it consists entirely of row upon row of Coca-Cola bottles. Someone must have been impressed; the 1962 silkscreen sold for $2.09 million in 1992. Warhol also painted *200 Campbell Soup Cans*, one with 50 repetitions of Marilyn Monroe's face, another that consists of 42 repetitions of Jacqueline Onassis's face, and still another with 80 repetitions of a two dollar bill. My guess is that Warhol had a somewhat chaotic lifestyle and therefore found the repetition esthetically satisfying.

Examples of repetition are not a modern phenomenon, though. The technique is commonly seen in art as far back as the eighth century B.C. as shown in Fig. 9-4 of the Greek vase.

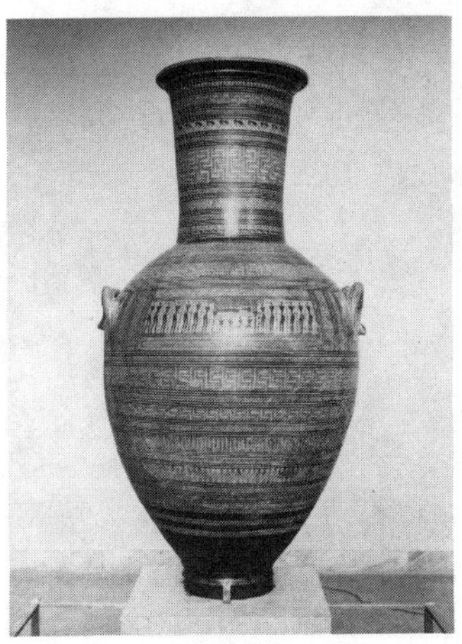

Fig. 9-4. *Dipylon Vase.* 8th Century B.C. National Museum. Athens.

Repetition has always been used in music from primitive drummers to the present groups. We've all heard rock music with such creative and inspiring lyrics as "Yeah, yeah, yeah, yeah, yeah, yeah;" "Oh, baby; oh, baby; oh, baby;" and the one that never fails to raise goose bumps, "I love you, I love you, I lo-o-ove you."

Repetition also occurs in architecture. My favorite example is the colosseum in Rome. But the epitome of repetition is reached in the glass boxes that serve as modern office buildings. In addition to their relatively low cost, the current popularity of such boring structures may be the balance they provide to the frenetic nature of the business world—and the world in general. Activities such as walking and jogging are the "glass boxes" of the exercise world.

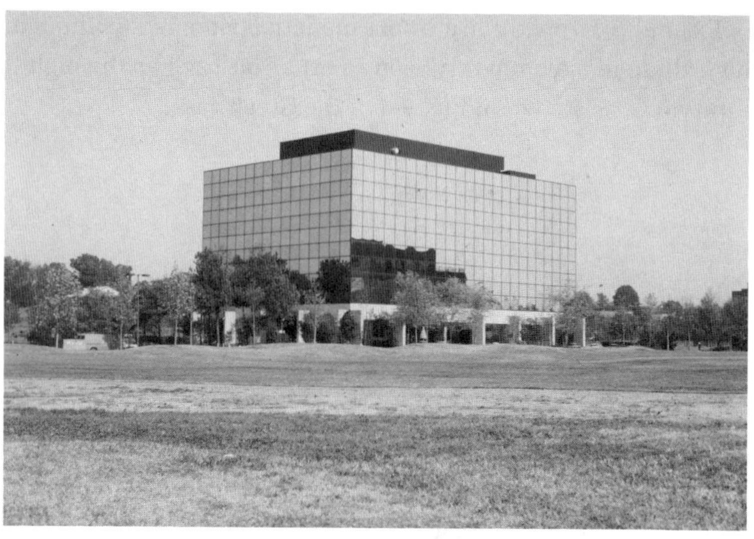

Fig. 9-6. A Basic Glass Box Building.

Some modern architects and their clients prefer structures that are visually more interesting than boxes with row upon row of glass panels. It's fascinating to travel through practically any city and look at the various glass-panel structures to see how principles of design and form are used to achieve increased interest. The variations range from slight modifications of the box to those that are almost dizzying in their complexity.

The simplest and most common way to make basic glass box structures more interesting is to separate each row of horizontal panels with a wide strip of concrete or other construction material.

The same effect is achieved, kinesthetically, when a person alternates 50 yards of jogging with 50 yards of walking. For a more interesting program, the walking can be replaced with different kinds of activities. The Swedes developed a popular exercise program called the Vita Course, based on this principle. In it a person jogs for, say, 50 yards. Does 10 push-ups. Jogs for 50 yards. Does 10 pull-ups. Jogs for 50 more yards. Does 20 sit-ups (curl-ups), etc. Many American cities have devoted space in their parks for such programs. As the architect of your exercise sessions you can use some of the same techniques used in buildings to create artistic kinesthetic structures in your repetitious exercises.

RESISTANCE EXERCISES

10

Resistance training is similar to calisthenics except that it uses equipment such as barbells, dumbbells, and various machines to increase the resistance to movement. The advantage of such programs is that tension in the muscles can be increased far more than with calisthenics, thereby leading to more rapid gains in strength. Resistance training also creates a greater range of body music because large variations in resistance can be quickly and easily achieved.

Esthetically, there could be a problem when the number of repetitions ("reps") is considered. People who want to quickly build large muscles should lift relatively heavy weights and do no more than five repetitions per set. Now, that is no problem kinoartistically because most people have the capacity to handle this number of elements.

But many people, particularly women, are instructed to do 10 or more reps—and 20 or more is not unusual. These numbers make sense if a leaner look is one's goal. But eight reps (elements), at the most, are more than a person can generally handle, intellectually or kinesthetically. Obviously there is a dilemma here between physical and esthetic goals that could make bodybuilding boring, or even unpleasant.

Fortunately, the dilemma is easily resolved by using the laws of esthetics in creative ways. As a simple example, assume you plan to do 15 repetitions of arm curls. You can divide the total number of curls into five smaller groups of three reps. During the momentary pause between groups you might take an extra deep breath or another breath. The pauses are periods of restraint or relaxation, which add interest to the kinoart. The pattern clearly will be more interesting than 15 identical repetitions.

Further, the number of groups and the number of reps in a group, can be varied considerably. For example, within a set of 15 there could be three groups of five reps instead of five groups of three reps. Of course, the number of reps per group need not be identical. When doing 15 reps, I sometimes do five reps (take an extra breath), do four reps (extra breath), do three reps (extra breath), do two reps (extra breath), and finish with one rep. If I'm feeling particularly macho, I'll continue by reversing the order and do one rep, then two, three, four, and five reps. That last set of five is rough. The climax, though, really captures my attention.

The most effective number of sets and repetitions for developing muscles is not "carved in stone." What works for one person may not work for another. And what works for one person may stop working after a few months. A lot of trial and error is necessary to get either optimal gains in strength and size—or leanness. Even though the most effective number of sets and reps may vary, kinoartistic methods can make every weight training program more appealing and exciting.

Bodybuilders are often reluctant to rest between groups within a set because the pauses greatly reduce the burning sensation in their muscles. These people are not necessarily masochists; most are merely students of the "no pain, no gain" school. They think medicine has to taste bad to be good for them. These devotees of pain think the "burn" causes faster muscle development.

That belief, however, is completely unfounded. The burning sensation is caused by lactic acid building up in the involved muscles. It accumulates because there is not enough blood flow in the muscle to carry the acid away. You see, the flow is diminished, or even cut off completely, when a muscle contracts forcefully. During relaxation periods blood flow increases dramatically. If there is not sufficient rest between reps, though, lactic acid accumulates and produces the burn. And research clearly reveals that lactic acid buildup does not stimulate muscle growth.

It is the *tension* within a muscle that stimulates growth. When lifting a weight, the tension is increased and the stimulus for growth is increased. Increasing the poundage will increase the tension—and the stimulus for muscle growth. A faster movement can also increase the tension—and the stimulus for growth. That is why sprinters have large muscular legs, compared to distance runners.

Lactic acid actually interferes with muscle development. As the acid level increases, it interferes with the ability of the muscle fibers to contract. As a result, the tension that can be developed by the muscle is reduced—and the stimulus for growth is reduced.

So, a relaxed pause after every repetition, and a longer pause after several repetitions, makes sense for physiological *and* esthetic reasons. The pauses allow blood to gush through the resting muscle and remove lactic acid and carbon dioxide (and bring in oxygen and sugar for energy). If you concentrate, you can actually feel the acid being drained away.

Even if there were no physiological advantages, the periods of restraint would be valuable in adding interest to an exercise. The periods help to reduce the number of elements to a level that can be easily grasped, intellectually.

I'm not suggesting that bodybuilders should avoid the "taste" of lactic acid. True, it does not help them build muscle tissue, but a sprinkling of the acid can add spice to a kinoartistic recipe. And if you are a masochist, go right ahead, stuff yourself with the stuff. Currently there is no evidence that a lactic acid buildup is unhealthy.

Bodybuilders are generally more in touch with their body music than any other type of athlete. After all, the lifting of a weight is a very personal endeavor, and bodybuilders, unlike other athletes, do not have to think about hitting, kicking, or catching a ball (or opponent). They do not have to react swiftly to changing strategies. Because their exercise movements are uncomplicated and can be performed slowly, bodybuilders can devote their full attention to each contraction of a single muscle or muscle group. They do not have to think about anything except their body music.

In a revealing and eloquent statement, the authors of *Pumping Iron: The Art and Sport of Bodybuilding* describe a Mr. Universe while he performed arm curl exercises as exhibiting an almost mystical concentration while focusing deeply within his muscle fibers.

The Mr. Universe was obviously in intimate communication with his body music. You may imagine him as being a rather strange fellow. But if you get involved in bodybuilding, you'll probably find yourself falling in love with each body part for about 8 seconds at a time as you exercise it—if you do it right. This may sound a bit narcissistic because, well, it *is* a bit narcissistic. But, there's nothing wrong with being a little in love with your muscles, as long as it's not too obvious to others and it's platonic.

Without a doubt a delightful kinesthetic "high" can be achieved in weight training programs *if* you concentrate on the sensations. Unfortunately, the sole desire of many weight trainers is to develop their bodies and get stronger. These people work out strictly as a means to an end. Future goals are important, not the exercises themselves. This attitude leads to boring experiences.

In *Muscle: The Confessions of an Unlikely Bodybuilder,* Samuel Fussell wrote:

> *I had to vary the exercises to keep from going completely insane. Lifting is more than demanding. It is fundamentally boring. Each day you know exactly what you are going to do, so you incorporate new techniques or movements, however minor, to keep from counting staples in the walls or numbering the tiles on the ceiling.*

Bodybuilding does not have to be fundamentally boring. Instead, a person should concentrate on his or her body music. If you are a kinoartistically oriented bodybuilder, you'll go one step further, though. You'll choose movements and organize them thoughtfully so exercise sessions will conform to esthetic ideals. Once the elements, designs, and patterns of practice sessions are formulated, attention can be given to the kinesthetic sensations of the movements. And due to the simplicity of bodybuilding exercises, you can devote a lot of your exercise time to giving your kinoart intellectual and emotional content.

If you are a beginning kinoartist, you should experiment by lifting light, medium, and heavy weights for each exercise—and concentrating on the kinesthetic sensations. You'll probably prefer the middle range. Light resistance will create barely discernible sensations. On the other hand, with extremely heavy weights, you will be keenly aware of the kinesthesia but it will tend to be unpleasant.

Unlike a novice, if you are an experienced bodybuilder you will often receive the most satisfaction from attempting to lift a very heavy weight. When successful, you will have the pleasure of fulfilling a very difficult kinesthetic type.

A good way for a bodybuilder to begin creating a kinesthetic pattern is to select a weight that can be lifted rather easily on the first repetition. An increased effort with each succeeding repetition will be perceived. Variety can then be added in terms of contrasts, complexity, and balance.

The simplest way to vary balance is by changing the width between the hands on the barbell. A narrow grip, for instance, will have the least degree of balance. One reason why weight training machines tend to be more boring than free weights is because the balance factor is eliminated.

Although it's impossible to make a drawing that accurately captures the qualities of kinesthesia, a crude visual representation of a kinesthetic experience can be shown with the series of vertical bars in Fig. 10-1. Using arm curls as an example, the thinner the bar, the greater the speed of movement; the darker the bar, the more intense the kinesthetic sensations of contractions; and the taller the bar, the greater the range of movement, etc. Spaces between bars could represent periods of restraint.

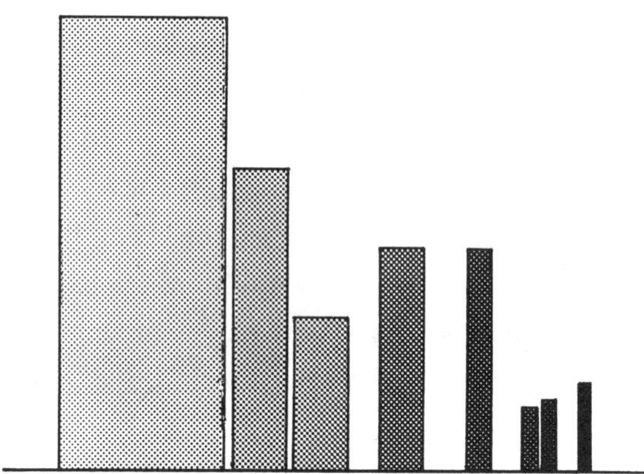

Fig. 10-1. A Visual Representation of Kinesthesia.

Of course, bars do not come close to capturing the richness of muscle kinesthesia. Besides, very few movements of the body are limited to just one muscle group. Nearly always, many other muscle groups must contract to stabilize other parts of the body.

A more realistic and complex kinesthetic pattern involving the superimposing of several muscle groups might well be visualized as Marcel Duchamps *Nude Descending Stairs*. Its different shading, colors, and shapes could well represent different muscle groups and durations and intensities of contractions.

Any one of thousands of paintings could have been chosen to illustrate the point. However, Duchamps was selected to appeal to the prurient interests of those who feel the spice of nudity improves the flavor of a book. I apologize to others who feel the painting is excessively titillating.

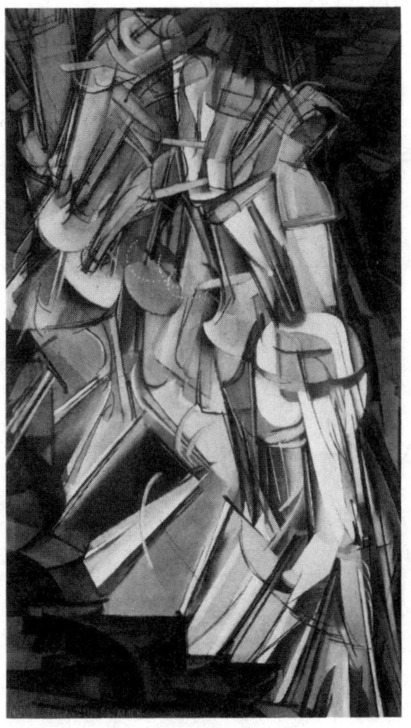

Fig. 10-2. Marcel Duchamps. *Nude Descending Stairs.* 1912. Philadelphia Museum of Art.

Additional ways to give kinesthetic variety to weight training are shown in Fig. 10-3 using the bench press exercise with a barbell. With a little imagination similar variations can be applied to other resistance exercises. Several position variations are shown. An extended pattern can be created by doing three repetitions in each of the four positions for a total of 12 repetitions. Slanted boards for doing incline and decline bench presses produce even greater differences in the quality of body music.

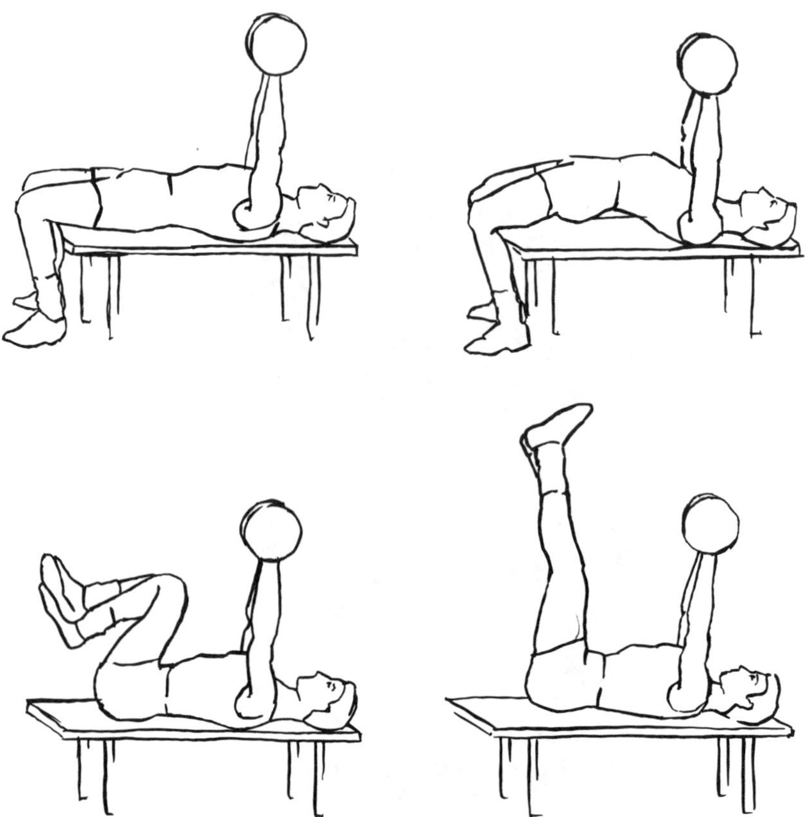

Fig. 10-3. Position Variations for the Bench Press.

Movement variations can also be created by pressing the barbell halfway up (four times), then all the way up (four times), and again halfway up (four times). Another pattern can be created by pressing the barbell halfway up (four times), then from the halfway position to full arm extension (four times), and finally four complete bench press movements. In all these examples the idea of related contrasts increases the kinesthetic interest of the exercises.

Further body music diversity is created when you press the barbell upward and then move it toward a position over your head (Fig. 10-4) or toward your feet—if the weight is very light. For safety these movements must be extremely slight, perhaps even hard to see. And you must have a spotter. Together, the movements produce a kinesthetic extension pattern.

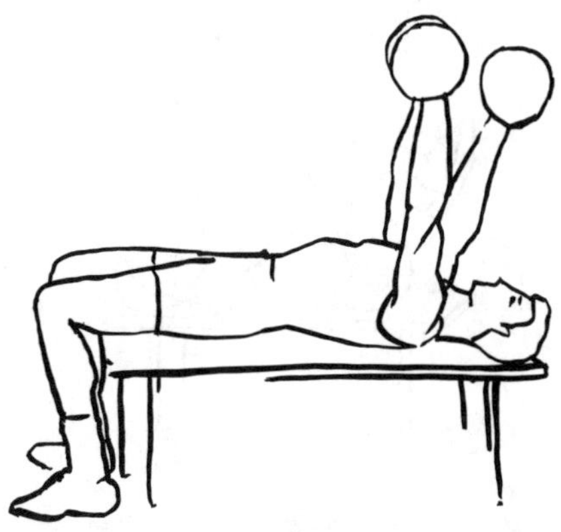

Fig. 10-4. A Kinesthetic Extension.

Because each exercise is different, variations for each may be different. With arm curls, for instance, I like to rock my body from side to side after each repetition, or after every two or three reps. With leg curls (that's where you lie face-down on an exercise bench and bring your heels toward your buttocks) I sometimes lift my elbows to the side in a single flapping motion, or I'll do an arm curl motion after each leg curl. These are all examples of kinesthetic extensions—if you concentrate on your body music.

Of course, kinesthetic sensations from other parts of the body can also be superimposed upon those of bench pressing. One way to do this is to extend your legs as depicted in Fig. 10-5 while pressing the barbell upward. If the kinesthesia of three presses are visualized as shaded bars (A) and the kinesthesia of the leg extensions as jagged lines (B), the superimposed pattern can be represented by (C). Just as the superimposition leads to a more interesting visual pattern, so is the kinesthetic pattern more interesting—infinitely more so.

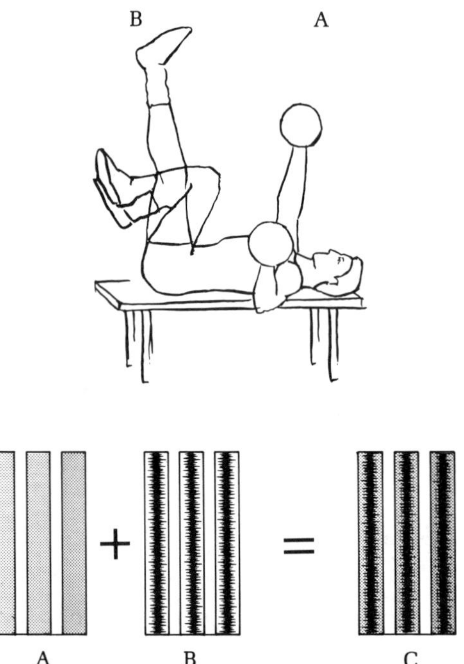

Fig. 10-5. Superimposing the Kinesthesia of Leg Extensions on those of Bench Presses.

Compared to barbells, dumbbells can produce a much greater diversity of body music because both arms do not have to move in unison.

Using the arm curl exercise, you can alternately move one hand at a time. That is, the left hand will move up and down—then the right hand will move up and down. Or you can lower one hand while simultaneously raising the other. Both exercises, incidentally, are asymmetrically balanced patterns which are more kinesthetically interesting than the symmetrically balanced patterns you are restricted to doing with barbells.

If you find arm curls to be boring, try bringing the dumbbells only one-fourth of the way up (and hesitate), continue to halfway (and hesitate), then continue to three-fourths of the way up (and hesitate), and finally bring the weight all the way up before lowering it to the starting position and doing a complete curl.

Another way to create contrasts is to change the kinesthetic quality of each arm curl. Fig. 10-6, on the next page, shows how this is done simply by rotating your wrists 90° after each set of three repetitions to create variations-on-a-theme. A gradation pattern can be created by gradually rotating the wrists during the lifting and lowering phases. Both of the these techniques, besides increasing the esthetics of the arm curl exercise, develop the elbow flexor muscles more fully.

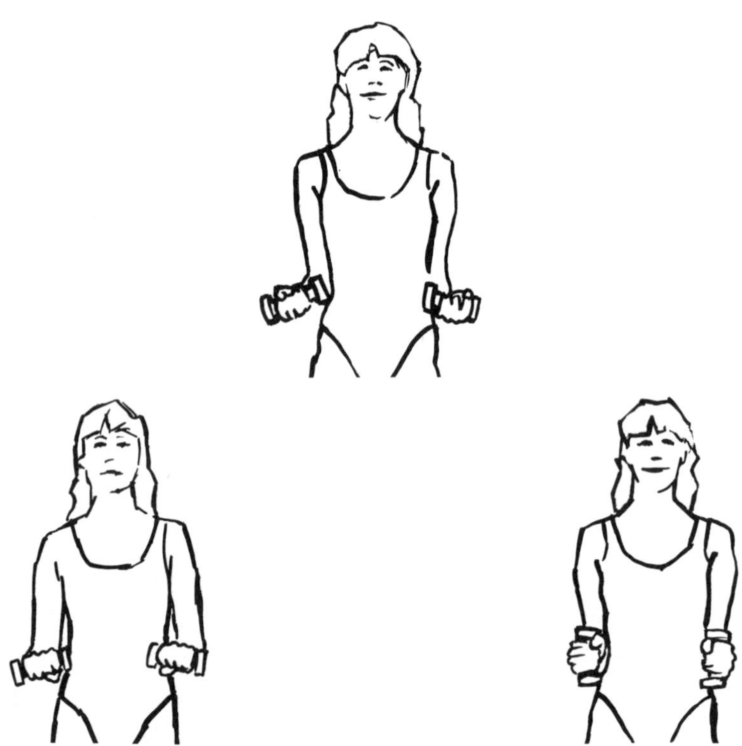

Fig. 10-6. Changing the Kinesthetic Quality of Arm Curl Exercises.

You can also shift your feet and turn your body 90° after each repetition, rock from side to side, or walk in place while doing arm curls. Superimposed kinesthesia from the lower part of the body makes for more complex and more appealing body music.

Shifting from front arm curls to lateral arm curls (Fig. 10-7) produces dissimilar contrasts in body music. You can also alternate the two kinds of curls, or gradually progress from one kind to the other. A combination of these two variations creates interesting out-of-phase circular motions (Fig. 10-8). Of course, the circular motions can also be done in-phase.

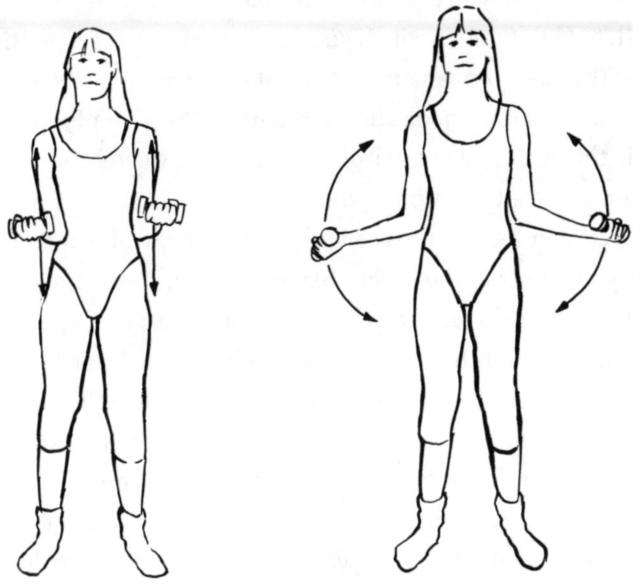

Fig. 10-7. Front Arm Curls and Lateral Circular Arm Curls.

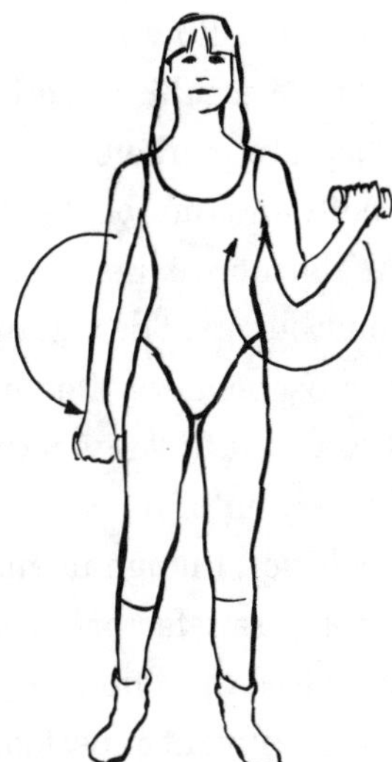

Fig. 10-8. Out-of-Phase Circular Motions.

If you find repetitions of any exercise to be boring and unpleasant, it is up to you to enliven the exercise. No one else knows what will be satisfying to you. If you enjoy doing a set of repetitions using just the basic movement, then do it that way. You needn't get fancy just because this book shows you how. Do what pleases you. After all, the major objective of kinoart is to liberate you while you exercise—not to restrict you.

I never let my designs and patterns control me; that would be silly. I control them. For example, I'll sometimes start a set intending to do nine reps in groups of three (with a pause between groups). If after the first three my body music is starting to "sound" really good, however, I'll omit the pause. I'll continue until I have trouble concentrating on the sensations (usually about five) or continue until the reps become unpleasant due to the buildup of lactic acid. At that point I'll pause, take an extra breath, and continue. If I'm feeling particularly macho, I'll accept the challenge that lactic acid hurls at me and triumph over it. In the end I always win because I am creating satisfying body music. Anyone can do it.

Many exercise machines allow the user to add resistance to exercise movements. These machines sell like "hotcakes" for a number of reasons. They are marketed much more aggressively than free weights (barbells and dumbbells) because a much larger profit can be made from the more expensive devices. Surprisingly, the high cost attracts some buyers. These people apparently believe an expensive machine must be more effective than a simple set of inexpensive weights. Besides, intricate workings, gleaming chrome, and shiny vinyl can be very enticing.

Most resistance machines, though no more effective than free weights, *can* give the user a satisfactory workout. A major disadvantage with machines is that they are usually boring to use. This is why people who have significant experience with machines and free weights almost always prefer free weights.

Free weights allow a wider variety of movement. The diversity adds excitement to exercising—especially if the weights are used properly. Like a marriage based solely on glitz and glamour, exercise machines are usually soon neglected—and shortly after—divorced and relegated to the attic or garage.

The main problem with exercise machines, as far as kinoart is concerned, is that the user usually does not get much kinesthetic variety. An analogy is a painter who has only one color on her palette. While some fine works can be produced by a master, as demonstrated by Picasso during his blue period, the artistic limitation does lead to boredom. It must be recognized, though, that boring exercises may be just what you need, just as the repetition of walking or jogging may be very attractive.

If you do find exercising on resistance machines to be boring, you, as a kinoartist, can do a lot to increase their kinesthetic appeal. For starters, organize the repetitions and sets of the exercises so they conform as much as possible to the laws of esthetics. Further, even when "locked" into a position so only the elbow can move (as shown in Fig. 10-9), you can change the body music associated with the exercise by varying the range of movement and by varying the tension in the muscle group. This can be done with changes in either the speed of movement or weight on the machine.

The person in Fig. 10-9 is not as locked-in as you might imagine. He can extend his legs while he extends his arms if he wishes and produce a superimposed combination pattern. Even if his body were completely constrained, he could create a vast number of body music compositions, isometrically, merely by pressing against the constraints or by simultaneously contracting opposing muscles.

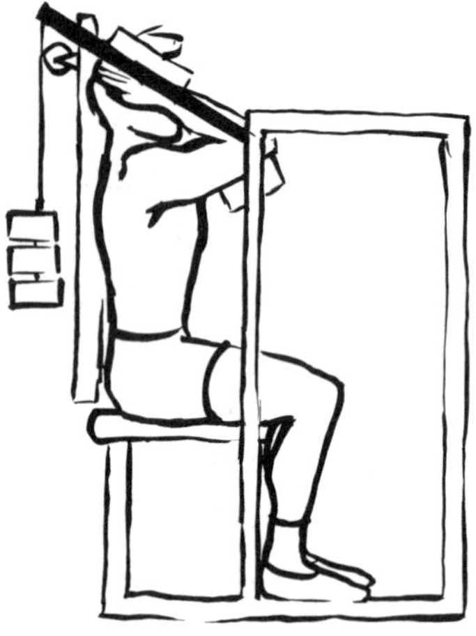

Fig. 10-9. An Exercise Machine that Limits Motion to Arm Extension.

Most exercise machines do not restrict movement to one joint if you use them creatively. The woman in Fig. 10-10, for example, can lean back as she extends her legs and lean forward as she flexes them (or vice versa). Or she can sit erect for four reps, lean back about 45° for four reps, and lie back for four reps.

In the latter position, to protect your back, make sure you keep the small of your back pressed against the bench; supporting your upper body with your elbows drawn back directly under your shoulders is helpful. With a little ingenuity you'll discover many ways to increase the richness of your body music while using machines.

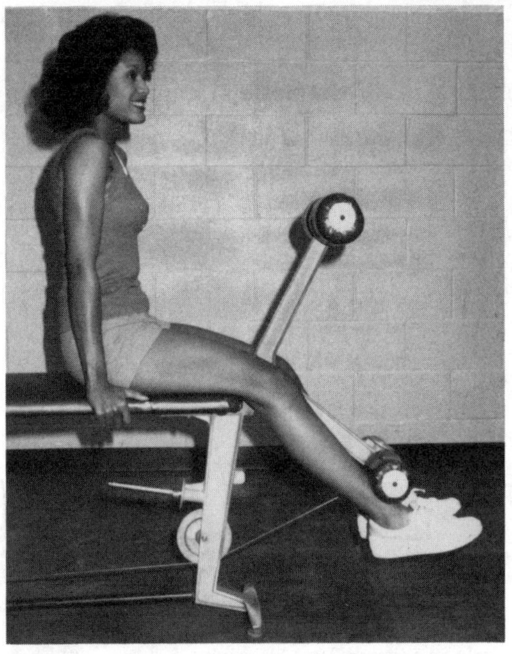

Fig. 10-10. Using a Leg Extension Machine.

A creative way to increase variations with machines is to use them in ways they were not designed to be used. The man in Fig. 10-11 has pushed the bench away from the bench press machine and is using the machine to do arm curls. From (A) he can bring his body to a slight forward lean while he curls the bar up to (C). Then he can lean back as he lowers the bar to (A). By allowing his body to move he has superimposed the body music from stretched muscles in his lower leg and ankle onto the body music of the curling motion. The total composition is thereby made more interesting than it would be with curling movements alone.

To make the exercise still more exciting, the man can lean forward and back between curling motions as shown in (E to A) to create an extended combination kinesthetic pattern. The kinesthetic sensations and rhythm of this arm curl exercise can be thrilling. Well, not as thrilling as swimming among sharks in a feeding frenzy . . . but a whole lot safer.

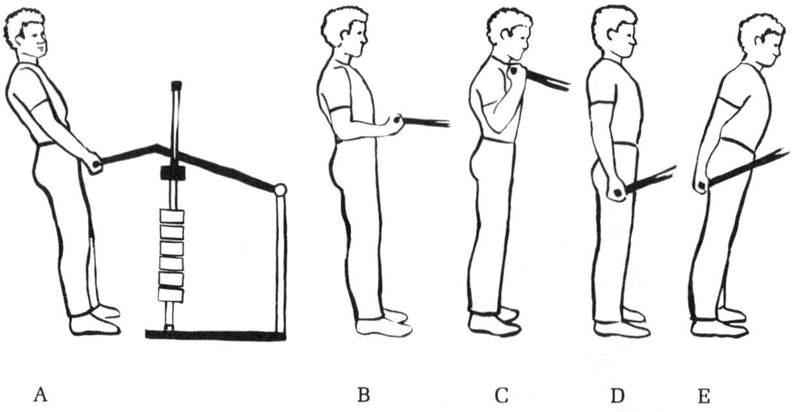

Fig. 10-11. Arm Curls on a Bench Press Machine.

Machines do have one distinct advantage over most free weights. You can rapidly and easily change the resistance. An example is the leg extension machine previously shown in Fig. 10-10. The simplified kinesthetic pattern visualized in Fig. 10-12 (with the shading of the bars indicating intensity of effort) is created when the woman extends her legs eight times with 10 pounds, six times with 20 pounds, four times with 30 pounds, twice with 40 pounds, and once with 50 pounds. She can then reverse the process and go back down the scale to 10 pounds. The kinesthetic pattern shows the slightly longer periods of restraint between the groups of repetitions to permit the changing of resistance. Besides being an arousing kinoartistic event, this kind of exercise pattern has a built-in warm-up. It also has both strength and endurance benefits.

If you choose the right weight, during the last few reps your leg muscles will be screaming for mercy. Umm, boy, that's fun! Seriously, some people *will* find the intense sensations very appealing. If you do not, don't worry about it. We all march to different drummers.

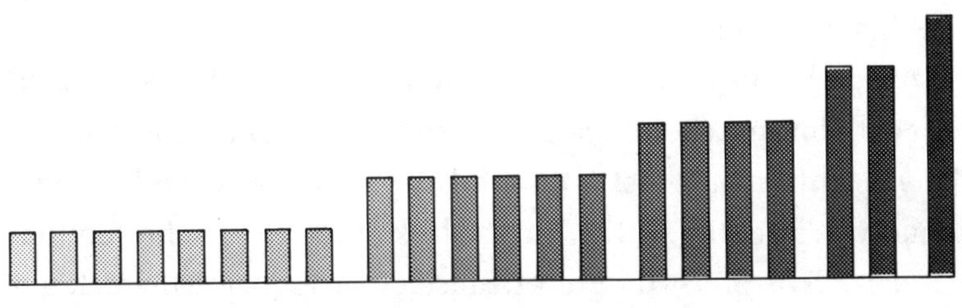

Fig. 10-12. A Visual Representation of the Kinesthesia Associated with the Leg Extension Exercise.

You do not need machines or weights for resistance exercises. Push-ups are an excellent example of how you can use your own body weight to increase resistance. Lunges and knee bends (pliés for ballet dancers) are other examples.

In fact, you don't even need to use your body weight. You can pit one muscle group against another. That was the idea behind the Charles Atlas Dynamic Tension Program. If you believe the advertisements, the Atlas system helped many a skinny lad develop big muscles and rise from humiliation to kick sand in his antagonist's face (and win back his fair lady). At one time, that heartwarming story graced the back cover of practically every comic book.

An example of dynamic tension is the "I must" exercise. Every teenaged girl knows the complete name. The exercise works equally well for both genders in strengthening the pectoral muscles. Begin the "I musts" by putting your hands together in a praying position, with your wrists in front of your forehead. Press your hands together for a few seconds. You can perform 10 repetitions without moving your hands. More than likely, though, you'll prefer to rhythmically move your hands up and down in front of your chest. More interesting kinesthetic variations involve moving your pressed hands from side to side, diagonally, in circles, or a combination of motions.

A big advantage of dynamic tension exercises is that you can do most of them anywhere, even while sitting in a car or in a meeting. Many people moan that sitting all day "broadens the bottom." Actually, it's not the sitting, but the lack of activity by the "bottom muscles." To exercise the gluteal muscles, just squeeze them. Right away, you'll notice the action lifts you in your chair. It might be prudent to do these exercises slowly. If not, you'll look like you're riding a trotting horse. If you contract the gluteals more slowly and one side at a time, you'll appear to be riding a walking horse. While both movements are fine types to kinolyze, they may cause colleagues to look at you askance. Or it may start a trend.

Repetitions in any resistance exercise, clearly, can be arranged to create body music that is more esthetically appealing than traditional resistance programs such as those consisting entirely of three sets of ten repetitions. As with all other art, however, kinoart is even more exciting when it has intellectual and emotional content. This is not as difficult as you might imagine. The first step is to simply decide on a type.

As Samuel Fussell revealed in *Muscle: Confessions of an Unlikely Bodybuilder,* the method is not uncommon at all among more experienced bodybuilders. He wrote:

> *I'd been at it for a full hour, painfully isolating my soleus and gastrocnemius muscles. To really 'get into them,' I was, of course, using the usual visualization procedure, in this case seeing my calves as gigantic spinnakers close to bursting from the force of a raging sea squall.*

Fussell speaks of "visualization." You should take that one giant step further. To use Fussell's example, instead of visualizing to "see" your calves as gigantic sails, try kinolyzing to "feel" how the sails would feel, kinesthetically, if they were near the bursting point. You will learn that the concept of kinoart is not merely a philosophical one, it's practical—and mainly, it's fun.

I started lifting weights when I was 19 and in the U.S. Marine Corps. For some reason I started varying the number of sets and repetitions to discover patterns I found most appealing. Of course, the concept of body music never occurred to me at the time. All I knew was that I liked the way my muscles felt when I lifted weights.

It took me years to realize it was the kinesthetic sensations of weight training that "turned me on." I was also boxing at the time, which I liked even more—a lot more. Much of that pleasure, I now realize, was due to boxing's rhythmic aspects. It was like dancing—a lot better than dancing actually, because in boxing you dance with your hands *and* your feet. Of course, in boxing you don't kiss your partner after the dance. As my coach was fond of saying, "When a fight's over, son, huggin' is okay, but no kissin'." He thought that was really funny.

The use of simple body music techniques probably helped my bodybuilding progress. I won the Mr. Heart of America physique contest (1958) a year after being honorably discharged from the Marine Corps.

However, far more substantial evidence of the value of kinoart is the fact that I am still training with weights and enjoying it 37 years after winning the contest. Over the years I earned a Ph.D. in exercise physiology (with a "minor" in psychology). I've taught those subjects and many others including anatomy and physiology, kinesiology, physics, biomechanics, and motor learning. Less formally, I've spent countless fascinating hours studying art history and philosophy. I've also engaged in a wide variety of athletic activities including tennis, dance (adagio and ballet), circus skills such as juggling, handbalancing, and unicycling, and skydiving. Actually, I don't know if skydiving can be considered a sport. All I ever did was close my eyes and jump—and pray.

I'm not revealing all of this background information to show you how wonderful I am . . . well, maybe a little. Mainly, though, I'm suggesting it was a unique mixture of academic, athletic, and artistic activities that gradually opened my eyes to the immense potential of body music.

For years I have experimented with applying various disciplines, particularly esthetics, to physical activity. This chapter and others suggest some of the many ways you can make the kinesthesia of exercise more enjoyable—and, therefore, exercise itself more fun. As an aspiring kinoartist, however, you should experiment to expand on the examples I've given. That's the best way to meet your own individual interests. It's also the way to find the most enjoyment. It is well worth the effort.

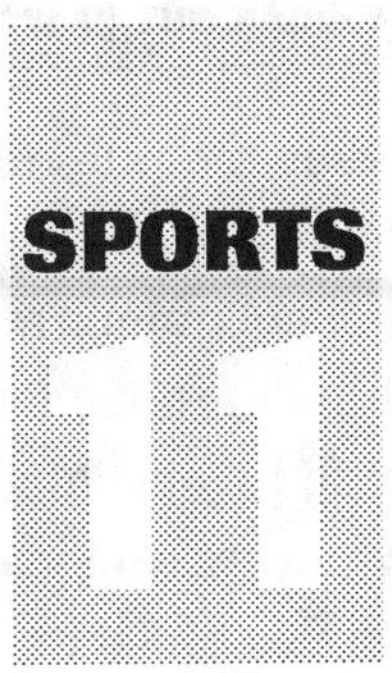

SPORTS 11

Sports are competitive physical activities that have a specific set of rules. Examples range from basketball and equestrian events to judo and sailing. Some sports such as gymnastics, skating, and diving are similar to developmental exercises (jogging, calisthenics, and weight training) because they allow participants to plan their routines in advance. Such athletes may even plan their movements to create specific kinoartistic patterns. Of course, gymnastics, skating, and diving are much more complex and difficult than developmental exercises. This complexity makes them far more rewarding when the routines finally are mastered.

In most sports, athletes have to instantaneously adapt their movements according to changing situations. Participants must concentrate on excelling at such activities as hitting, throwing, kicking, jumping, and running. During competition the associated kinesthesia is, by necessity, a secondary consideration. Nevertheless, the movements in sports can produce extraordinarily complex and beautiful body music. Whether an athlete is aware of them or appreciates them is an individual matter.

Athletes do not have to be merely observers of their kinesthetic sensations and hope they will be appealing. In spite of the movement limitations imposed by the rules of each sport, athletes can still have considerable control over their kinesthetic patterns.

Esthetic limitations are not unique to kinoart. Movie directors must practice their art within the boundaries of a script, musicians have boundaries determined by each composition, and portrait painters are restricted by the appearance of their subjects. (Okay, someone forgot to explain that to Señor Picasso.)

It's a waste of time and effort for artists to complain about the restrictions imposed by a script, composition, or rules of a sport. It is better to consider restrictions as challenges and then wisely devote energy to a more fruitful area—overcoming personal limitations of creativity. Success will come to those who develop and perfect their techniques through contemplation and practice.

The techniques of a kinoartist involve the control of his or her joint movements and muscular tensions. And although most athletes cannot plan all their actions, there is much they can do to improve the esthetic appeal of their body music. The key is to train so their movements are biomechanically sound.

The science of biomechanics applies mechanical laws to human movement. The main laws deal with balance, the development of forces, and the dissipation of forces. When commentators speak of an athlete's mechanics, they are referring to how well he or she is adhering to the principles of mechanics. How closely athletes obey the laws determines how well they play their games.

Incidentally, the reason many people do not enjoy playing sports is that they're not proficient at the activities. That's true for children as well as adults. If all physical education teachers and coaches based their instruction upon biomechanical principles, students would become proficient more quickly and be far more likely to find enjoyment in physical activity. As Thomas Shadwell wrote in 1679 in his play *A True Widow*:

Every man loves what he is good at.

Even more to the point is a statement by J. Bronowski in his book, *The Ascent of Man.* He said for every practical action there exists pleasure, simply in the action for its own sake. Further, *the pleasure that humans find in perfecting their skills is responsible for every work of art.* The aim of kinoart, of course, is to help people obtain maximal pleasure in the practical action of exercise.

Having sound biomechanics not only affects athletic performance, but also the esthetics of body music. For example, when a batter swings at a ball, the movement tends to feel good kinesthetically, even when he misses it—*if* his movements were biomechanically correct. Of course, he shouldn't merrily explain, "I struck out again, Coach, but the swing sure felt delightful!"

Conversely, the batter may get a base hit but experience unsatisfying body music—if his swing was biomechanically unsound. Generally, though, if a movement feels good kinesthetically, it means the movement was biomechanically correct and the athletic performance was more likely to be successful. In other words, there tends to be a direct relationship between an athletic performance and its kinesthetic appeal.

The relationship is so close that an athlete should devote time and effort to becoming more kinesthetically aware. As George Sage states in *Introduction to Motor Behavior,* a book about learning physical skills:

> *There is little doubt that kinesthetic perception is important to the performance of motor skills.*

Kinesthetic concentration should be stressed during all practice sessions where the learning of movement skills are involved. Unfortunately, this is rarely done.

Once the kinesthetic sensations associated with good biomechanics are deeply ingrained, athletes can shift more of their attention toward the competitive aspects of their games. In the long run, kinoartistic involvement is not inconsistent with sports' traditional aim of winning. On the contrary, such involvement helps athletes perform more successfully.

In competitive games it is easy to understand why people would devote all of their attention to winning. This intensity can have negative effects, however, when carried to the extreme. As sociologist H. Roy Kaplan has said in his lectures:

> *Fueled by excessive competition for the elusive win . . . sports are becoming devoid of humanism, cooperation, esthetics—even enjoyment.*

You probably know players who endure unpleasant and harmful levels of emotional stress when they compete in sports. If they lose, they are crushed. Their day is ruined and those around them are also forced to suffer. Even when they win there are invariably times throughout the contest when they are dissatisfied with the score or their performance. They shout and curse, or slam down equipment in frustration and anger. In the "big business" of professional sports where winning so often is everything, perhaps such behavior can be understood. It certainly has no place, however, in recreational events where enjoyment is the chief aim.

Ironically, an obsession with winning often has an adverse effect by causing players to "choke," forget strategy, or waste energy. On the other hand, it is very difficult to be hampered by a "must-win" attitude when players devote some of their attention to their body music. Logically, the less competitive an activity is, the more a participant can concentrate on moving in a kinesthetically pleasing way.

The body music approach to sports actually helps people refresh the mind and body far more easily than the "win at all costs" approach. Players with this recreational attitude can never lose. While they may end up on the short end of the score, which should be irrelevant to them anyway, they will have created a satisfying and rewarding work of kinoart.

In play there are two pleasures for your choosing—
The one is winning, and the other losing.

Lord Byron. *Don Juan,* xiv

Some coaches believe practice has to be arduous, oppressive, and grim. If players smile or look like they are having fun, they are berated for not taking the workout seriously. (It is, after all, a *work*out.) These coaches believe medicine has to taste foul to be beneficial. It is virtually impossible for coaches with this philosophical stance to use kinoart in their practice sessions.

On the other hand, there are coaches who do not believe players have to be treated harshly and inhumanely. These coaches view their athletes as sensitive, intelligent humans and will be receptive to the idea of planning practice sessions that are founded, in part, on esthetics. They will recognize the value of helping their athletes develop kinesthetically. Not only will the players find practice sessions more enjoyable, they will also learn physical skills more readily and, therefore, perform better in competitions.

Athletes who wish to become kinoartists can begin by developing an awareness of their body music. It's suggested they follow the procedures in Chapter Seven (exploratory exercises). Then they can progress to the skills required in their sports. They should begin with slow movements and with a minimum of distractions, such as opponents, to better concentrate on their body music.

It is also important that a knowledgeable coach helps athletes improve the biomechanics of their skills so the proper kinesthetic rhythms will be remembered. Once the kinesthetic sensations of a movement become deeply ingrained, the movements will tend to feel right even if they are based on poor mechanics. At that point it will be very difficult for an athlete to learn the correct mechanics because its associated kinesthesia will feel strange and disturbing.

A softball batter is used here as an example of how kinesthetic awareness can produce positive results in a competitive sports program. First, a batter should stand at the plate and swing the bat without a ball being involved at all. This way he (or she) can devote his entire attention to the body music of the batting movements. Again, a coach should instruct him on the proper mechanics. For instance, to effectively use the forces produced by his muscles, a batter begins by stepping toward the ball. As his foot touches the ground, his rear foot pivots to allow his hips to rotate; then his trunk and shoulders rotate. Next his arms extend, followed by rotation of his wrists. For a properly executed sequence each motion must flow from the preceding one so the individual forces are added smoothly. This results in the bat traveling fastest at the moment of contact with the ball.

At first the batter should perform the movements slowly, and then increase them to full speed. As always, he must *concentrate* on the associated body music, particularly the rhythm of the sensations, so the kinesthesia of a well-executed swing will be remembered. Performing the swing with his eyes closed is particularly effective.

After a batter has kinesthetically grooved his swing, he should start practicing with a batting tee (Fig. 11-1). In this situation he must hit the ball, but because it is stationary he can still give considerable attention to his kinesthetic rhythms.

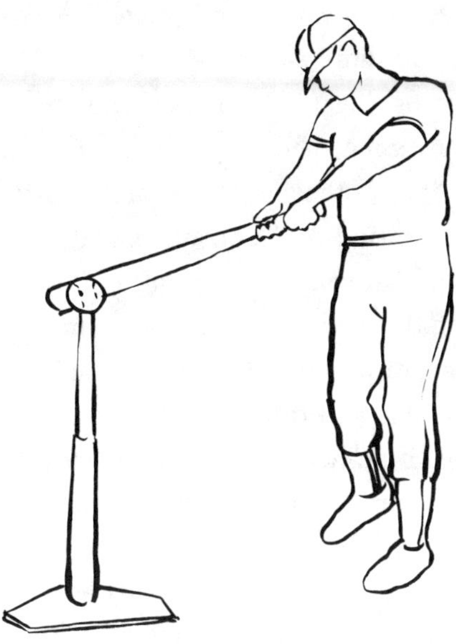

Fig. 11-1. Using a Batting Tee to "Groove" the Kinesthesia of a Swing.

When a player can consistently hit the ball with power and accuracy from the batting tee and still feel the body music of his swing, he can then have a pitcher throw the ball to him. A pitching machine is even better because it is has better control. In either case, the ball should be thrown slowly at first. Gradually the pitching speed should be increased until it reaches competitive levels. Not a lot of time should be spent on the lead-up phases. It is the body music of a normal, full-speed swing that a batter wants to become imprinted on his or her mind.

When an athletic skill, such as batting, is based on kinesthetic patterns, it can be repeated over and over with little or no loss of effectiveness. A kinesthetic imprint allows players to more intensely enjoy the batting experience. It also makes them better hitters because a consistent kinesthetic pattern logically should help eliminate batting slumps.

The body music compositions associated with sports have the potential to be much more satisfying than those of calisthenics, weight training, or jogging. First, sports permit more diversity and spontaneity of movement because they are less formally structured. Because their kinesthesia is more complex, their body music is richer and more exciting. A visual representation of the kinesthesia of batting a ball, for instance, would surely be closer to Prueitt's Computer Generated Drawing than to the paintings used to represent the kinesthesia of weight training and jogging. Second, compared to the resistance and repetitious activities, the kinesthetic types in sports are far more difficult to achieve. When successful, therefore, the efforts are much more rewarding.

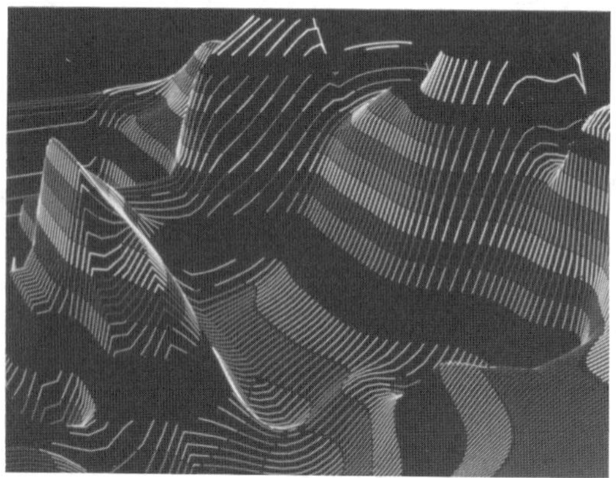

Fig. 11-2. Melvin L. Prueitt. *Computer Generated Drawing.* Los Alamos National Laboratory. Los Alamos, New Mexico.

In sports the simplest types are determined by the nature of each sport. That is, the types are synonymous with immediate goals. For a quarterback, a type might be a successfully thrown pass. A type for a golfer might be a long tee shot straight down the fairway.

Goal-oriented types do not mean athletes cannot have kinoartistic experiences while playing sports. They often do, even when they know nothing about kinesthesia. Edmund Vance Cooke was years ahead of his time when he wrote in *Prayer*:

Perhaps the reward of the spirit who tries,
is not the goal but the exercise.

A similar sentiment is voiced in an ancient Chinese proverb:

It is not the destination that is important.
It is the journey.

So often one hears an athlete say how beautiful and effortless a movement felt, whether it was a pole vault, shot put, or dive. More often than not, the movement will have been successful in fulfilling a type. That is due to the positive relationship between skill and kinesthetic patterns.

DANCE

12

Performance dances such as ballet, modern, tap, and jazz are athletic events that are often more difficult than sports. Ballet, for example, has been estimated to be more demanding than any sport in terms of total physical fitness—the components of which include balance, flexibility, strength, speed, power, endurance, agility, and neuromuscular coordination. In addition to athleticism, the beauty of a dancer's movements is judged by spectators, choreographers, or critics.

In the ancient Olympic Games, judging for grace was involved in all events; now it is considered in only a few sports such as gymnastics, diving, and skating. In most sports it does not matter how graceful an athlete's movements look, as long as he or she strokes a base hit, sinks a basketball, or scores one for the Gipper.

Performance dances and body music are intimately related. In both art forms, esthetic designs and patterns are created through body movements. The major difference is that dancers create artistic visual images while kinoartists are absorbed with creating artistic *kinesthetic* images.

You can be a dancer and kinoartist at the same time, though, because a dancer's visual expressiveness is closely related to body music. Similarly, if you are moving in a visually beautiful manner, your body music will likely feel beautiful, also. This explains why some dancers get greater pleasure in dancing without an audience. The applause is missing, but without the necessity of pleasing other people they are free to concentrate more intensely on the beautiful kinesthetic sensations created by their movements.

Choreographers often exhort their dancers to:

Make your movements say something!

Dancers must constantly strive to communicate meanings and arouse feelings in an audience. When a prima ballerina portrays a dying swan, the audience should be inspired to empathize with the swan type and feel sorrow. A hula dancer relies on the stylized motions of her hands to express intellectual types and emotions.

How can you put meaning and feeling into a performance? The tables on page 87 give just an inkling of the relationship between movement and feeling. The list is far from exhaustive. Otto Harbach, an American playwright, was right on target when he observed that every little movement has a meaning all its own, and that every thought and feeling may be shown by some posture. It is common knowledge that a person's emotional state is reflected by his or her posture, gait, gestures, and facial expressions.

One does not need psychological training to tell if another person is feeling depressed, exuberant, angry, or whatever. Words are usually not necessary. In fact, words are often deceptive. It's easy to lie with words. Not so with body language.

Early in the 1800s the French diplomat, Talleyrand, said:

Speech is a faculty given to man to conceal his thoughts.

And who would be more aware of this than a diplomat.

Not only do emotions affect body postures, but the reverse is also true. Body positions and movements—or more accurately, the associated kinesthetic sensations—affect emotions. Walking erectly, for example, gives a person more self-confidence. And the mere act of smiling, even if you do not feel like doing so, makes you feel more positive about yourself and others. And it actually makes healthy physiological changes within the body.

The immense possibilities for variety of expression is revealed by the gesture language of the classic Hindu dance wherein 57,000 *hand* positions have a distinct meaning. This should be an especially heady number to people who, consciously, use only a single gesture—a finger gesture, and an obscene one at that.

Even though dancers communicate with an audience on a visual level, they can and must be simultaneously communicating with themselves on a kinesthetic level. Each form of communication serves to reinforce and enhance the effectiveness of the other. More specifically, if you feel an emotion, kinesthetically, you will be much more successful at conveying that emotion visually. This is why choreographers constantly urge their dancers to:

Try to feel your movement.

Though it is never too late to begin, kinesthetic awareness should be stressed at a dancer's first lesson and continued through every subsequent lesson. Further, dancers should kinolyze whenever possible to heighten their portrayal of roles. To use the dying swan example again, when kinolyzing a dancer should attempt to feel the kinesthesia of the injured swan as it slowly and painfully dies. This technique cannot be overemphasized; it is the height of kinoart and it greatly enhances a dancer's performance.

It is not the intent of this book to teach you to dance. There are already many philosophies and methods of dance instruction. The sole purpose of this section is to help you use body music to make your performance (1) kinesthetically more appealing to yourself and (2) visually more appealing to your audience. The task should not be difficult since dancers' movements have already been painstakingly preplanned (choreographed) with esthetics in mind. All that remains is for dancers to concentrate on their body music.

The first dance lesson should always begin with a person learning the most basic and most important dance skill—good posture. It is probably impossible to improve on Martha Graham's delightful description of good posture. She said it was the instant of apparent stillness when the body is poised for the most intense, most subtle action, and is at its moment of greatest potential efficiency. Clearly, good posture is important not only for dancers but for everyone.

A balanced standing position depends on the proper alignment of the various parts of the body. When body parts are properly aligned (Fig. 12-1), a vertical line through your body's center-of-gravity will (when viewed from the side) pass just behind the ear, through the shoulder joint and hip joint, and continue in front of the ankle. A common suggestion is to pretend a string is tied to the top of your head and someone is pulling upward on it.

That's not a bad idea. Most people find the advice very helpful, but you mustn't let your shoulders "hunch up." Keeping the neck long gives the impression of "lightness." As you practice this posture you should, of course, *concentrate* on how it feels, kinesthetically, so you can reproduce the position. A fun experience is to kinolyze what an ostrich or giraffe would feel as it extends its head upward to its full height.

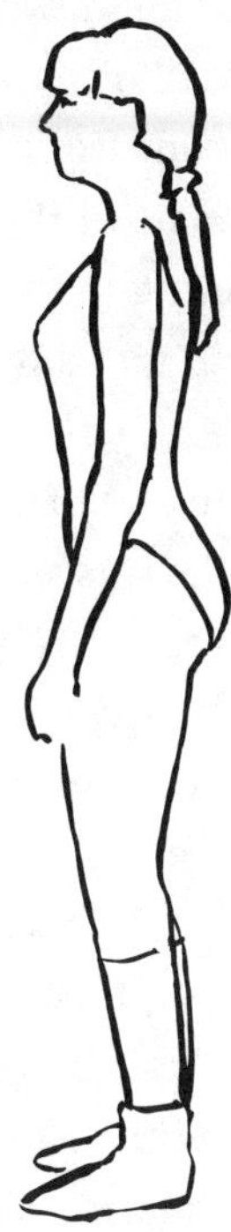

Fig. 12-1. Proper Alignment of the Body for Good Posture.

Initially, it will be very helpful for beginning dancers to use a mirror to check their posture. They cannot rely on kinesthesia to tell them if their body is properly aligned. After years of poor posture, its kinesthesia will feel correct and that of proper alignment will feel incorrect. With practice, not just in the dance studio but throughout the day, the kinesthesia of good body alignment eventually will feel "right."

With good alignment you can explore the movement possibilities of the torso. Consisting of the shoulder, mid-section, and pelvic regions, the torso is the most fundamental segment of the body because it provides a base for movements of the arms, legs, and head. The torso is itself, however, capable of many movements. It can bend forward, backward, sideways, and rotate. The motions can be combined and different parts of the spine can even move in opposite directions—as anyone from Chubby Checker's "twist" era knows. That is, the lower part of the spine can rotate to the left while the upper part is rotating to the right. In addition, there can be further variations in torso movement in terms of the direction, range, speed, and quality (e.g., jerky versus smooth).

At the very least, the muscles of the mid-section must contract to stabilize the torso when the legs, arms, or head move. Normally, though, there is a far more active relationship between the torso and the extremities. Nearly always, an action will begin with movement of the torso and flow through the involved extremity. This is dramatically clear in activities requiring very forceful motions of the extremities such as a discus or baseball throw. In most daily activities, however, torso motion is more subtle. Even then, it is important not only for a more graceful appearance and more efficient movement, but because it gives a greater sense of body wholeness, or unity, in terms of body music.

For instance, when you walk without any torso motion, you will kinesthetically perceive the movements of the arms and legs as two separate kinesthetic patterns with little esthetic appeal. However, when you walk with appropriate torso action, the body music from the torso muscles links the body music of the arms and legs to produce an integrated pattern that is perceived as an artistic kinesthetic whole.

John Wayne's distinctive way of walking, in which the entire body was actively involved, is a perfect example of a unified kinesthetic experience. If you want to have some fun, try and imitate it—and maybe it would be best to do it when not too many people are around. I have found that when I try to walk like the Duke, people tend to treat me a whole lot differently. Or maybe it's just my imagination.

If you really want to have fun, try moving like Tina Turner; it might be best to do it in private, especially if you're a male. And try not to hurt yourself. At the same time *concentrate* on your body music and you'll experience a kinesthetic smorgasbord.

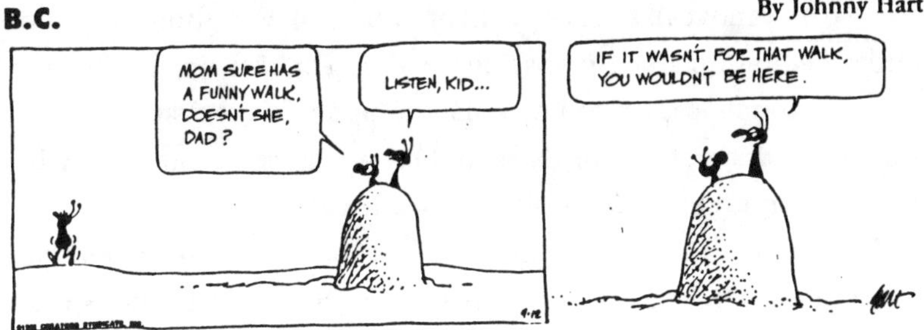

B.C. by permission of Johnny Hart and Creators Syndicate, Inc.

The mastery of proper body alignment is not desirable for stationary positions alone. You should also maintain proper alignment while moving. As soon as you have a clear kinesthetic perception of proper standing posture, you should slowly begin shifting your body weight from side to side so it falls on one foot and then the other. The next stage is to barely lift the heel of the free foot as you rock from side to side. Gradually the height of the foot is increased until the toe is barely off the floor. Then you should slowly walk in place and begin swinging your arms in opposition to the legs. Next, begin to slowly walk forward with very small steps, then ever larger steps until you are walking at a normal gait and with appropriate arm swings.

Progress gradually from one phase to the next, while always maintaining proper body alignment and kinesthetic awareness. As with sports, not much time should be devoted to the lead-up phases. It is the body music of normal walking that you want to become ingrained.

As soon as walking with good posture is mastered and its body music clearly perceived, you should advance to the more complex, more exciting patterns of running, skipping, hopping, leaping, jumping, galloping, and sliding—in all directions. There can be combinations of movements and combinations of directions so people may move in a curved path or even spin. Variations in speed and acceleration are also possible. Walking on tiptoes, flat-footed, or in a crouched position can also be done. Movements may be relaxed and swinging, or tense and stiff. The potential variety in locomotion is staggering—almost infinite.

The mastery of movement should not be limited to locomotive skills, however. You can remain in one spot and explore your space by reaching with your arms and legs. You can crouch low, lunge, kneel, or do pliés, pirouettes, and so on. Wearing a blindfold will really heighten the way you experience your kinesthesia. In every case, though, if a movement is to have full form, meaning, and feeling, you must *concentrate* on your kinesthetic sensations. This concentration is basic to the creation of kinoart (body music).

In performance dances, choreographers pre-plan movements to create visual experiences that are esthetically appealing to an audience. Some people mistakenly believe choreographers have the only creative role in dance and dancers are little more than mobile mannequins. However, a successful dance depends on a successful partnership between choreographer and dancer. A choreographer's task, in its simplest description, is to arrange movements that will be esthetically pleasing to an audience. A dancer's task is to give life to the movements so they will not seem mechanical, so spectators will perceive meaning and feeling in them.

You can do this most effectively by being keenly in touch with the body music associated with your movements. In other words, you should be feeling kinesthetically what you want the audience to perceive visually. If there is a discrepancy between the two perceptions, the performance will suffer. It would be similar to a performer who sings the gospel song "Amazing Grace" with fast, jerky body movements. Your ability to harmonize your body music with the visual sensations of the movements is what maximizes the sensitivity and quality of a dance composition.

There is a bonus with this kinoartistic approach to dance. So often a choreographer or instructor feels saddled by the chore of having to motivate his or her dancers. With kinoart, that task is eliminated. Dancers will not have to be driven because they will be so attracted by the wonders and delights of artistic kinesthetic patterns and designs. And this is no exaggeration.

In 1928 those sensations inspired a Hungarian named Rudolf Laban to develop a system of movement notation, analagous to music notation. The inspiration for Laban's ingenious work began when he was 15 years old and moved by an especially beautiful sunrise in the mountains. He wanted to express his feelings:

> *But how? In words, in music, in paint? But it was all too rich for that . . . I moved. I moved for the sheer joy in all this beauty and order, for I saw in it all. I saw something which is absolutely right, something which had to be so. And I thought, there is only one way I can express all this. When my body and soul move together they create a rhythm of movement; and so I danced.*

Without knowing kinesthetic sensations even existed, the young man became a kinoartist on the spot. Laban's reaction may seem strange to some people, but it is not at all unusual. Just watch practically any youngster who is excited for whatever reason. Some will express their feelings by frolicking about, shaking, etc. Children are natural kinoartists; they revel in movement.

You must strive for sensitivity in your movements not only during performances but at every practice session and rehearsal.

You should not perform even the simplest developmental or stretching exercises at the *barre* without concentrating on creating artistic kinesthetic events. As you practice your art, your body music will become more and more refined and beautiful. It is hard to imagine any motivation being as powerful, and this applies not only to dancers but to all kinoartists whether they are participating in bodybuilding, jogging, or sports.

FREE EXPRESSION ACTIVITIES

13

As the name suggests, free expression activities allow you to move as your spirit motivates. Your attention is not diluted by physical fitness goals, game rules, or choreography. You are completely free to move in any manner you wish. Since there are no limitations, free expression activities have the greatest potential for kinesthetic creativity and satisfaction. Because of the delightful sense of freedom, of being totally in charge of one's life, free expression activities should be attractive to people who feel stuck in the bureaucratic incarcerations that characterize our society. And there are millions upon millions of such people.

Sometimes called "improvisation" in the dance world, free expression activities may be performed on the spur of the moment for no other reason than to revel in the delightful feelings of body music. The activities may also be exploratory in nature to help you expand your kinesthetic horizons. The appeal of this type of kinoart may be founded solely on form (design and pattern), but it is virtually impossible to imagine a body music composition without some meaning and feeling attached to it.

Indeed, you may have an intellectual type in mind before beginning to improvise. An example of a type would be a golf ball rolling toward the cup. In this case you would try to feel and express the kinesthesia of the ball as if it had kinesthesia. That is, you would be kinolyzing. Understandably, the process may sound a bit strange, but it makes exercising far more fun and exciting. Try it; you'll like it. It does not take long to get the "hang of it." You may get so involved in kinolyzing, say, a salmon swimming up the Columbia River, that 30 minutes of otherwise boring swimming may seem like five or ten exciting minutes.

Kinolyzing involves more than pretending, although pretending is certainly involved. That reminds me of a cartoon in which a woman is riding a stationary bicycle. She's telling a friend that the only thing that keeps her pedaling is pretending to be going as far from the gymnasium as possible. The woman, of course, is pretending. While escape is not a lofty source of inspiration, it does give her activity the intellectual content it needs to "keep her going." It's better than nothing. If she would concentrate on her kinesthesia, she would have a far more positive experience. If she would kinolyze the kinesthetic sensations of a gazelle fleeing a cheetah, she would really improve her chances for an thrilling exercise experience.

Not everyone, of course, will find the same kinolyzations stimulating. With my instinctive good taste, I've selected the following cartoon to show how a typical young man might use kinolyzation to heighten the pleasure of riding a bicycle.

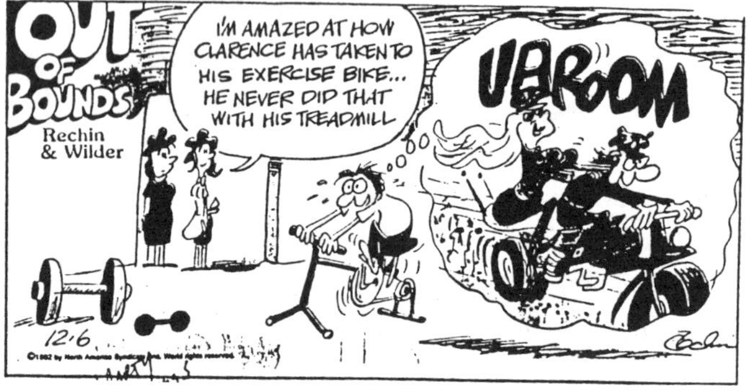

OUT OF BOUNDS (cartoon) by permission of North American Syndicate, Inc.

A stationary bicycle, incidentally, may not appear to offer nearly the potential for body music as does a mobile bicycle. But many movements which would be dangerous or impossible to perform on a regular bicycle, such as riding free-handed while doing trunk-twisters, can be done easily and safely on a stationary bicycle.

You may enjoy throwing punches while riding a stationary bike. You'll burn more calories; that's for sure. You can begin by throwing a jab every time a pedal descends. Begin with each fist in front of its shoulder. Have the palms facing each other. When the left pedal descends, throw the left fist straight out from the shoulder while rotating the left shoulder forward. At the same time rotate the wrist so the palm faces downward. Bring the fist back to the shoulder immediately. Then, when the right pedal descends, throw a right jab. Or you may want to pedal several times between punches.

There can be a lot of variety even if you only throw jabs. When you jab and push the pedal down as described above, the feelings will tend to feel harmonious. If you prefer more jarring sensations, try jabbing while pushing the opposite pedal down.

If you know how to throw hooks, intersperse them with the straight punches. A hook is a bit more complicated than a jab, but the complexity makes it a more exciting body music composition. Not many people know how to properly deliver a hook. Here's your opportunity to learn (that knowledge is sure to put joy in your heart). Begin with each fist in front of its shoulder. Have the palms facing each other. As the left pedal starts to descend, lift your left elbow and deliver the punch in a curved path toward your right shoulder. The palm should always be facing your body. The right hook is just the reverse of the left. Even without riding a bike, throwing punches is a delicious kinesthetic experience. Plus, we can be boxing champions without marring our pretty faces.

For a number of reasons I recommend that every household have a "heavy" bag to beat on. In less than a minute of "all-out" punching you will know why the activity is excellent for developing the upper body and cardiovascular system.

You have seen how kinolyzing can be used to enhance body music and give it meaning and emotion. Try to kinolyze yourself in the Olympic boxing finals; I have a whole drawer full of imaginary gold medals. You may even experience the sensations of a kangaroo who is "duking" it in a circus sideshow, or be one of the knights of the Round Table jousting in a medieval tournament. There is no valid reason for anyone not to try kinolyzation. It surely beats working out. And your wallet remains unmolested.

If you are a bodybuilder, you can pretend a barbell is a prison bar and you are straining to free yourself. Taking it one step further, you can imagine your kinesthesia as being that of a grizzly bear as you rip a tree trunk (barbell) overhead. Besides adding considerable content to the kinesthesia of weight lifting, such kinolyzing can help you exert more effort.

The woman in the *pas de deux* in Fig. 13-1 may be kinolyzing an airplane being catapulted from a carrier deck. Her partner may be imagining his body music to be that of a pilot.

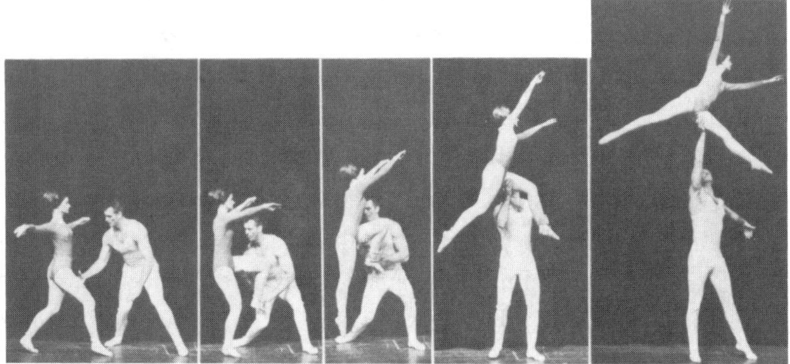

Fig. 13-1. A Lift in a Pas de Deux.

Before creating kinoartistic types with free expression activities, it's a good idea to first watch young children at play because so many of their movements represent types. When children see a picture of a train they merely recognize a rather common visual type. But when they "choo-choo" around the yard with piston-like stomps of powerfully driving legs and choppy to and fro motions of bent arms, they *become* the train.

Children typically kinolyze many types through their kinesthetic sense. And they would continue to do so as they grew older, if such behavior were encouraged. Unfortunately, because it is not encouraged, it is cast aside with other "childish things." Just as a child's scribblings, if continued, could lead to masterpieces and mud pies are the forerunners of fine sculpture, kinesthetic "choo choo trains" would surely lead to sophisticated and satisfying body music if such an activity were not "nipped in the bud." This is not to say a child's work of art cannot be as appealing and sophisticated as an adult's (even a respected artist)—as revealed in (A) and (B) of Fig. 13-2. Indeed, I think Cynthia's painting is better than Miró's.

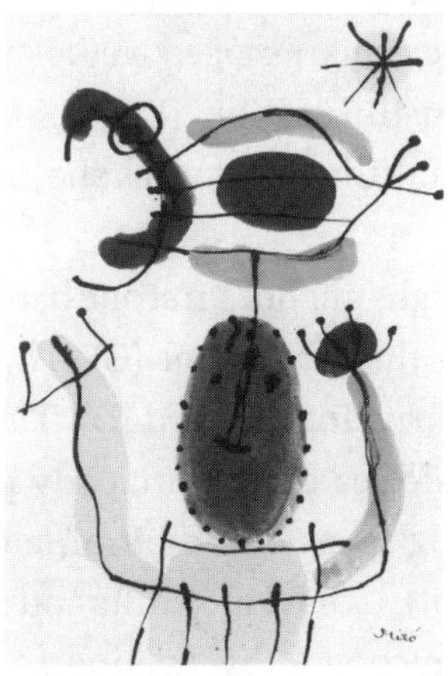

Fig. 13-2 (A). Joan Miró. *The Lyre Bird.* 1962. ARS, New York/ADAGP, Paris.

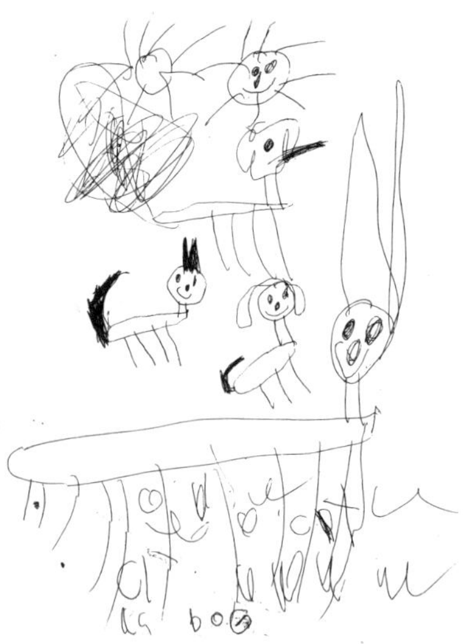

Fig. 13-2 (B). Cynthia Schroeder (age 4). *Cats.* 1974. Courtesy the artist.

Adults, if able to "let go," logically should be far more proficient than children at creating kinoart with intellectual and emotional substance. For example, a person may kinolyze a type that consists of a sailing vessel making an ocean voyage. One type of ship could be a large square-rigged vessel that, initially, is at anchor. In (A) of the illustration (Fig. 13-3) that follows, the woman's body music fulfills that type as she languidly sways from side to side.

When the ship weighs anchor, first one bank of sails is unfurled and trimmed (B) and then the other (C). The untethered vessel immediately begins thrusting forward (D). The woman expresses the effect of a moderate sea by rhythmically propelling her body forward with thrusting leaps and a bit of lateral motion (or she could stand in one spot). If the wind shifts and comes from her port (left) side, the ship responds by heeling to starboard (E). The woman may find the body music of lunging forward with her right leg to be even more meaningful (F).

As the wind freshens, the ship's plunging actions intensify. Then as the winds shifts again, the vessel heels to port (G). The plunging motions can be kinesthetically represented not only by lunges and movements of the kinoartist's entire body, but by deep inhalations and exhalations as well.

The woman's movements become more expansive and powerful as the gale strengthens. When hurricanes levels are reached, her arms begin to swirl violently about her head (H). Finally one arm goes limp (I) to kinesthetically portray a yardarm being broken and hanging useless. Then the other arm drops to her side (J). Her body movements become erratic as her rudder is swept away, causing her to rotate aimlessly. A reef is abruptly struck and the once proud ship shudders agonizingly and falls, crippled (L). The pounding seas drive her relentlessly up and down, up and down on the treacherous coral (M). The woman's push-ups (N) become progressively lower and slower. She rises more sluggishly each time as the ship fills with water. With a tortuous convulsion of her entire body, the ill-fated vessel rolls over and slips beneath the foamy surface. Only a broken mast is visible (O). Finally, it too is gone.

If this were a 10- to 15-minute "voyage," the kinoartist would probably want to remain on the "bottom" for a while to recover. She will have had considerable exercise because her voyage used all the muscles of the body, particularly the large muscles of the shoulder, chest, arms, and legs. However, due to its emphasis on intellectual and emotional content, this free expression activity is a vast improvement, kinesthetically, over a calisthenics program using the identical muscle groups. Clearly, this creative approach to exercise cannot be considered a workout—it is kinoart. a body music composition.

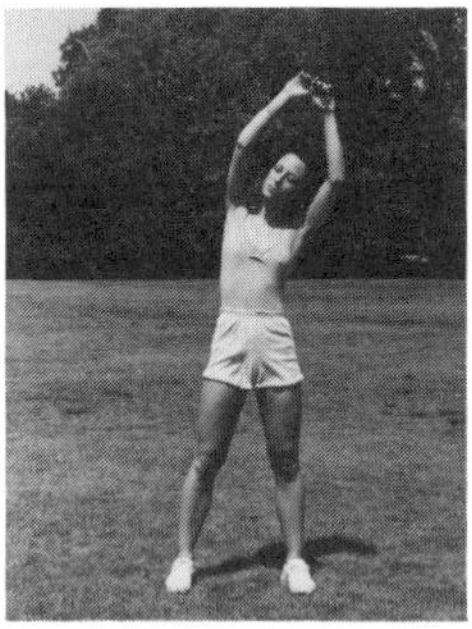

A 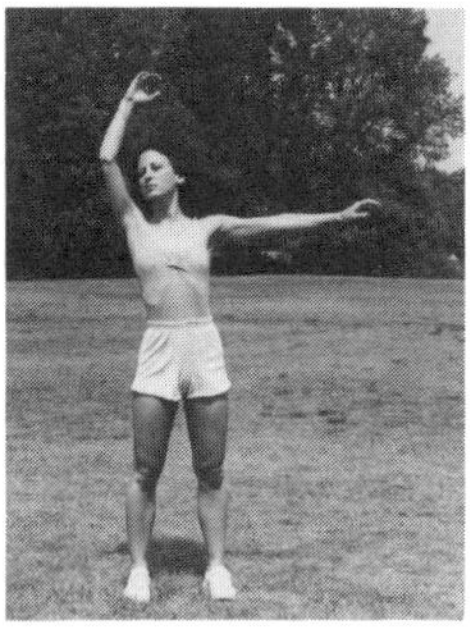 B 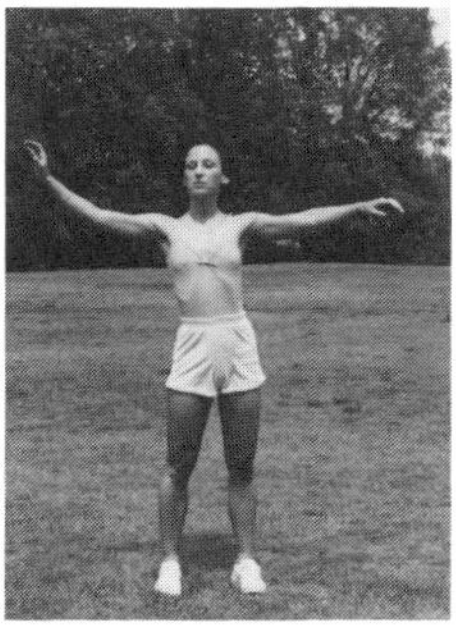 C

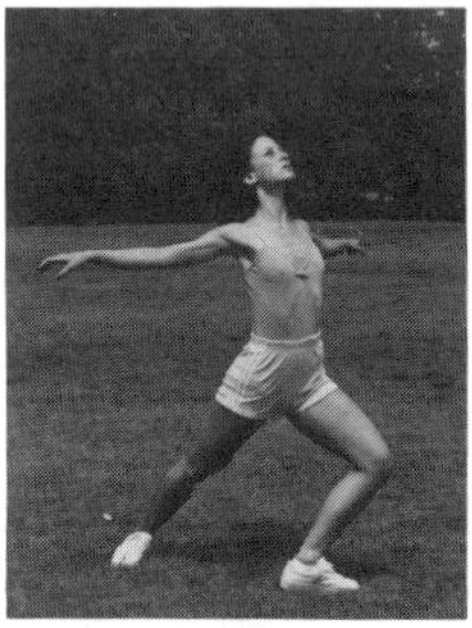

G 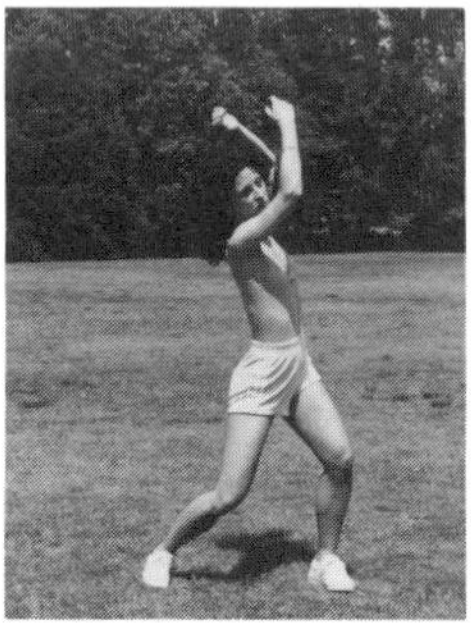 H 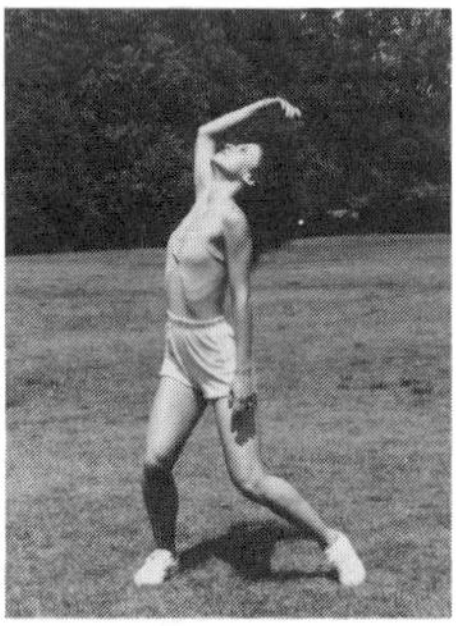 I

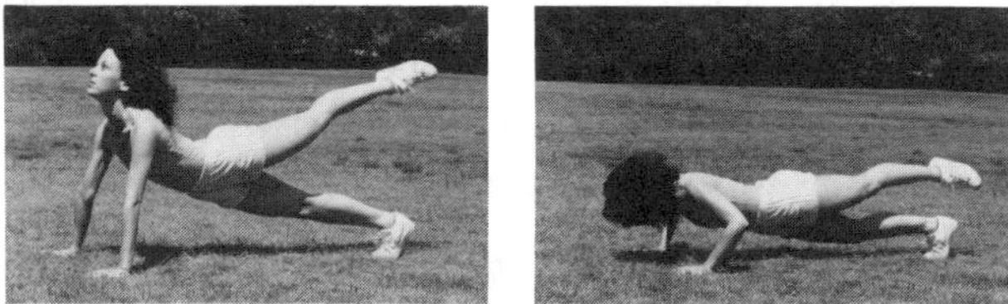

M N

Fig. 13-3. A Kinoartistic "Voyage" Created by Free Expression.

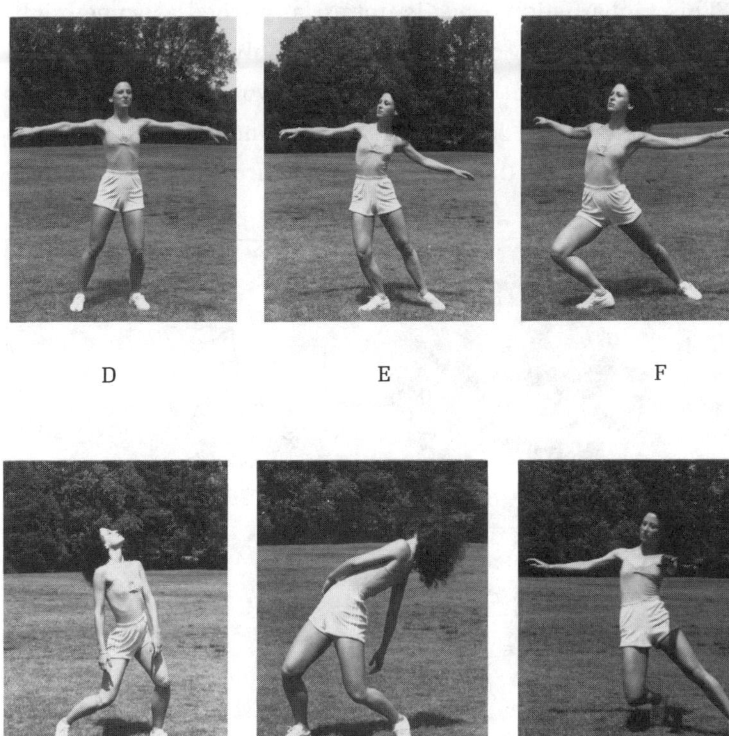

D E F

J K L

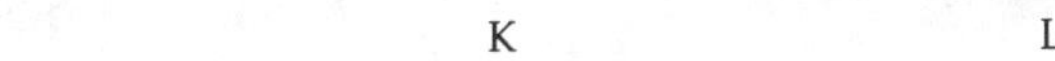

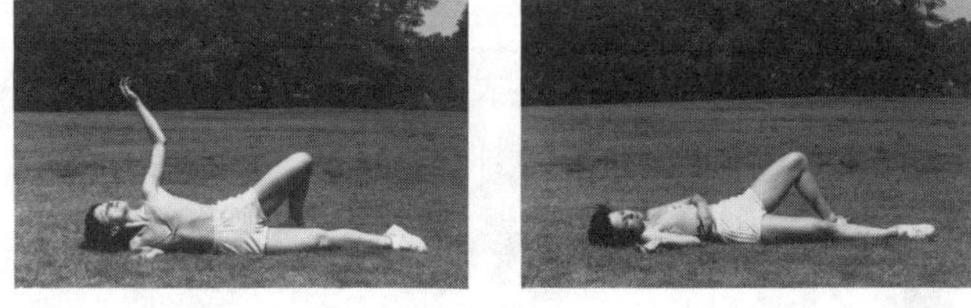

O P

This kinoartistic voyage is not as far-fetched as some might believe. The following cartoon is funny simply because of its truth. Practically every adult with even a hint of youth remaining in his or her heart has done something similar—and been caught in the act. With kinolyzing, though, you go a lot further by involving the kinesthetic sense.

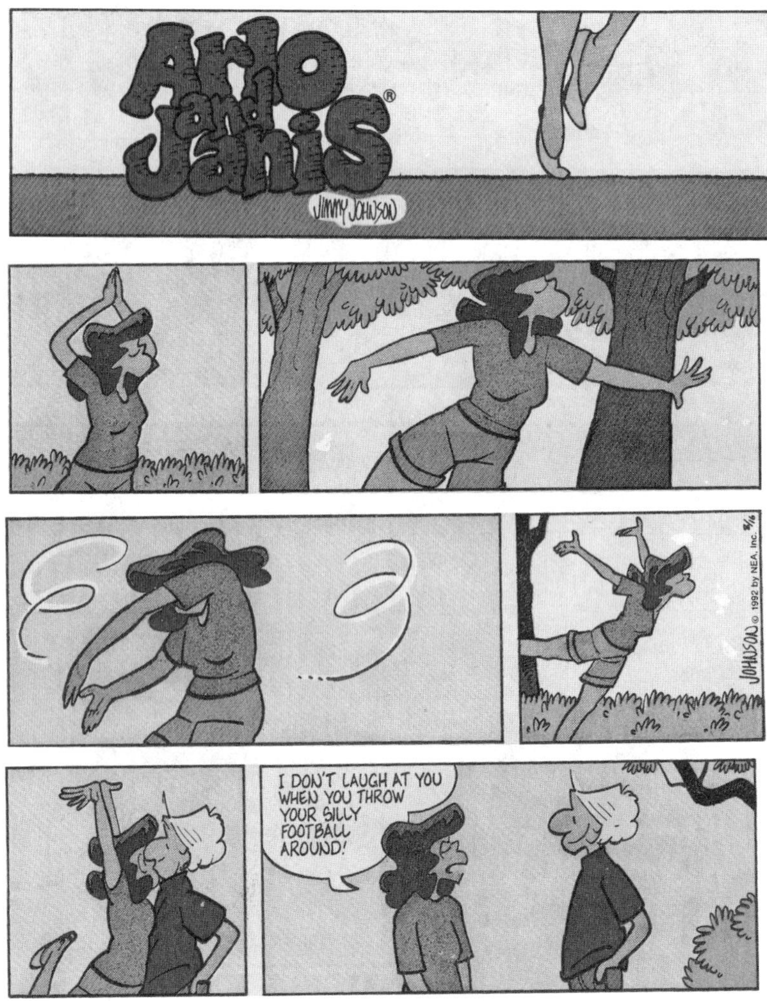

ARLO & JANIS reprinted by permission of NEA, Inc.

Among the most unique and exciting kinesthetic types are those created in the zero gravity of water. When you slip under the surface, you can undulate sinuously to create within your mind the kinesthetic image of a playful porpoise. You can dart and glide like a barracuda or streak upward from the bottom of the pool and break the surface like a hooked marlin. You are limited only by your imagination.

Wearing fins helps immensely in the creation of types because they allow you to swim faster and they free your arms. One interesting exercise is to swim while letting your arms drag behind. With the hands cupped in a relaxed fashion, experiment with a number of positions so that different sensations are experienced in the palms and fingers. In some positions it feels as if I am holding a handful of shaking Jello; it may feel a bit different to you. Try it. It will add a lot interest to moving through the water.

My favorite swimming type for kinolyzing is a submarine. As I swim with fins, my propeller shafts (arms) project backward alongside my trim, steely hull (that would be my body, of course). I am obviously a technologically advanced vessel. My propellers (extended hands) move slowly as I slip rapidly through the water in search of a worthy adversary, Red October, the pride of the Soviet submarine fleet. The natural pointedness of my bow (head) gives me a distinct advantage for running silent, running deep.

I do have a problem with the huge squadrons of mini-destroyers that invade the pool on weekends. These five- to twelve-year-old vessels swarm through the waters and occasionally collide with my sleek, handsome hull. I would love to sink a few of the pests, but their mother ships maintain too careful a watch. And those battleships have firepower—way too much—even for me.

The ultimate kinesthetic type, flight, can also be done in water. Unlike air, water *is* dense enough to support the human body. In water we can "fly" with the greatest of ease. Some people enjoy being kites or maple seeds being blown about. If the water is deep enough and you have a weight belt, adjust the poundage to alter your buoyancy and spread your arms to the sides and soar like an eagle or do aircraft maneuvers such as barrel rolls and loops or whatever. Extending your arms past your ears you can surface dive and rocket downward, swoop up to stall, and then lunge down again. Scuba tanks, besides visually and tactilely reinforcing the "jet" type, enable you to perform "aerobatics" for long periods while being totally immersed.

If it sounds as if I act like a "kid" while I'm playing in the water, I guess that's because I *am* acting like a kid. It makes sense because I feel youthful when I'm creating kinesthetic types. And for a person who will be 60 in a few years, the shedding of years may the greatest benefit of kinolyzation.

And remember, the physical benefits of exercise are not diminished at all with the body music process. The benefits are actually enhanced because activities are more fun.

Kinolyzing is more than just pretending to be a fish, plane, or submarine. Pretense is part of it, but the most important aspect is trying to feel the kinesthesia of those objects—as if, indeed, they all had kinesthesia. Such creativity is where the greatest challenge and enjoyment lie.

Kinolyzation may seem silly, but people would probably be a lot happier if they "lightened up" and were a bit silly now and then. Exercise, especially, needn't be a somber endeavor. Kinolyzation readily allows you to be a little silly and have fun while exercising. For this reason, of all the kinoartistic experiences you'll probably find free expression the most enchanting.

The number of kinoartistic types possible in free expression is limitless. In terms of *time*, a type can develop from a four-hour stint at the wheel of a tractor trailer to the brief period of weightlessness people experience when their vehicle speeds over the crest of a hill.

In terms of *effort*, type can be based on events varying from the lifting of a heavy weight to the graceful extension of an outstretched arm. In terms of *movement*, the body music of a sudden sprint can produce the image of a leopard's charge while the body music of riding a bicycle in sand can conjure the spirit of Michelangelo's *Bound Slave.*

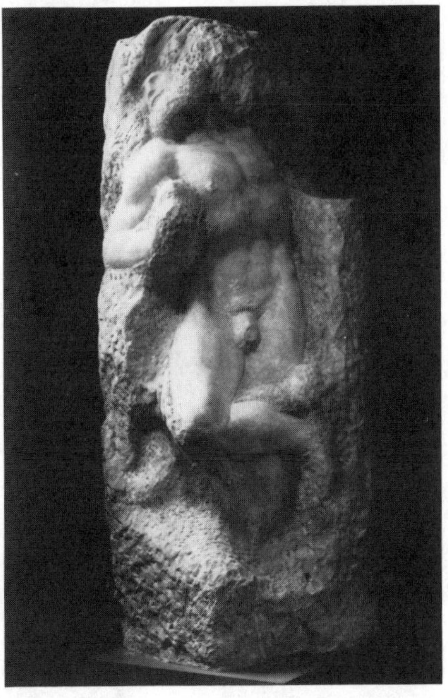

Fig. 13-4. Michelangelo. *Bound Slave.* Alinari/Art Resource, N.Y. 1519-20. Galleria dell'Academia, Florence.

You may understandably feel "funny" doing free expression exercises with other people watching. I sometimes do. In fact, when I plan to "close down" most of my mind and move spontaneously to concentrate on my body music, I make sure I'm alone. A few embarrassing movements might pop into my creations.

If you practice in private, embarrassment will be no problem. Kinoart is not a performing art, anyway. "Letting go" is the important thing. Along with concentrating on your body music, it is the foundation of free expression.

CONCLUSION

People who have some awareness of their kinesthesia are pleasantly surprised when quite by chance they recognize a pattern in those sensations. This compares to the delight of seeing a pattern in clouds or a splatter of paint that reminds them of something. These people have good imaginations, but cannot be called artists.

An artist produces sensory experiences that express ideas and arouse emotions. Whereas painters, musicians, and chefs deal with combinations of colors, sounds, and tastes, respectively, a kinoartist deals with combinations of kinesthesia. To create these combinations a variety of activities ranging from calisthenics, weight training, and jogging to sports, dance, and free expression can be used. Because kinoart, or body music, has intellectual, emotional, and esthetic dimensions along with physical benefits, it is vastly more satisfying and more enjoyable than merely "working out."

Kinoart produces a "rush"—a healthy, socially acceptable rush. It may not be addicting, but it surely is habit forming.

It's not always easy to create art, especially for a beginner. One recommendation for creating art was suggested by the English painter, William Turner. He had "no settled process" but:

> *. . . drove the colors about until I had expressed the idea in my mind.*

By substituting "kinesthesia" for "colors" the same advice can be given to a kinesthetic artist. Turner's method requires a lot of experimentation. A preplanned application of the principles of esthetics, however, would greatly reduce the time-intensive trial-and-error process. In any case, some study, thought, and practice is necessary to learn to arrange kinesthetic sensations into artistic forms that have intellectual and emotional content. The results, though, will surely justify the time and effort. As Oscar Wilde said:

It is through art, and through art only, that we realize our perfection.

Applying this idea to physical activity, it can be said:

It is through kinoart, and kinoart only, that the perfection of exercise is realized.

Speculation on the possibilities of what is yet to come in the realm of body music is most exciting. In just 66 years there was a transportation revolution as we advanced from a 12-second airplane flight to trips to the moon. Sixty-six years! Kinoart may well lead to a similar revolution in the approach to physical activity. At least the art form is now "off the ground."

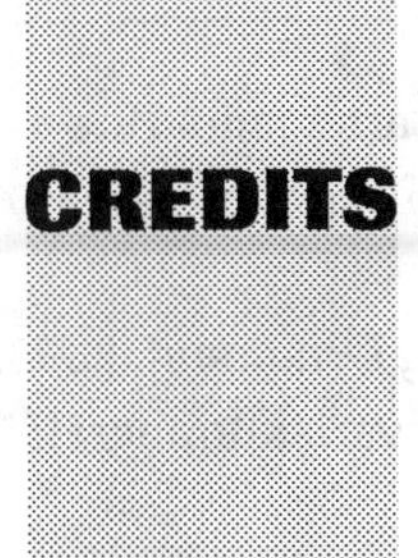

CREDITS

A wide variety of books, articles, photographs, and cartoons were used in this book. The author and publisher wish to express their deep appreciation for permissions to use all of the source material. In all cases, every effort was made to contact copyright holders. If there is any oversight, we will be eager to update our information.

There is no uniformity in the credit lines because different organizations require different forms when giving permission. Most of the credits, particularly for art and cartoons, are given in the text near the works. Some organizations require a credit line in both the text and in this section.

Page 41. Thomas Munro, *The Arts and Their Interrelationships*, The Press of Case Western Reserve University, Cleveland. 1967.

Page 45. Jackson Pollock, "*Autumn Rhythm*," Oil on canvas, 105 x 207. The Metropolitan Museum of Art, George A. Hearn Fund, 1957. (57.92).

Page 48. Francisco Goya, "*The Clothed Maja*." Museo del Prado, Madrid, Spain.

Page 51. William McCarter and Rita Gilbert, *Living With Art*, Copyright © 1985. Permission of Alfred A. Knopf

Page 70. *Viking Clothing Ornament.* 2096.24, Go, Viking era, Alva parish, brakteat, Antikvarisk-topografiska arkivet, Stockholm, Sweden.

Page 80. Piet Mondrian, "*Composition,*" 1929. Oil on canvas. 17 3/4 x 17 7/8 inches (45.1 x 45.3 cm) Solomon R. Guggenheim Museum, New York. Gift, Estate of Katherine S. Drier, 1953. Photo: David Heald, Copyright The Solomon R. Guggenheim Foundation, New York. FN 52.1347. Reprinted with permission.

Page 84. Horst de la Croix and Richard G. Tansey, *Gardner's Art Through the Ages.* Harcourt Brace Jovanovich, San Diego, 1986.

Page 115. Chuck Close, "*Self Portrait,*" Memphis Brooks Museum of Art. Gift of the American Academy and Institute of Arts and Letters, New York; Hassam, Speicher, Betts and Symons Funds 1991. 91.4.

Page 123. *Dipylon Amphora*, Greek. The National Archeological Museum, Athens, Greece.

Page 131. Samuel Fussell, *Muscle: Confessions of a Bodybuilder.* Poseidon Press, New York, 1991.

Page 151. George Sage, *Introduction to Motor Behavior.* Permission of Addison-Wesley Publishing Co., Reading, Massachusetts, 1977.

Page 173. Joan Miró, "*The Lyre-Bird,*" 1962. Gouache and china ink on paper. Private Collection, Paris. Photo supplied by Galerie Lalong, Paris. Reprinted with permission. (Although titled "The

Lyre-Bird" in art books, this was listed as "Untitled" by the supplying museum.)

Page 181. Michelangelo, *Slave*, Accademia, Florence, Italy. Reproduced with permission of Art Resource, New York.

BIBLIOGRAPHY

Every book proceeds from the information and inspiration of previous writings. In turn, it is hoped that the new book will provide a similar function for subsequent works. The author is particularly grateful to the authors of the books listed below.

Boggs, Joseph. *The Art of Watching Films.* Palo Alto: Mayfield, 1985.

Delaumosne, L'Abbe. *The Delsarte System.* New York: Edgar S. Werner, 1893.

de la Croix, Horst and Tansey, Richard G. *Gardner's Art Through the Ages.* San Diego: Harcourt Brace Jovanovich, 1986.

Ellman, Richard, ed. *The Artist as Critic.* New York: Random House, 1968.

Fixx, James. *The Complete Book of Running.* New York: Random House, 1977.

Fussell, Samuel Wilson. *Muscle: Confessions of an Unlikely Bodybuilder.* New York: Poseidon Press, 1991.

Gaines, Charles and Butler, George. *Pumping Iron: The Art and Sport of Bodybuilding*. New York: Simon and Schuster, 1974.

Hajek, Lubor and Forman, Werner. *A Book of Chinese Art*. London: Spring Books, 1966.

Hawkins, Alma. *Creating Through Dance*. Englewood Cliffs: Prentice-Hall, Inc., 1964.

Herrigel, Eugene. *Zen in the Art of Archery*. New York: Vintage Books, 1971.

Houston, H.P. et all. *Introduction to Psychology*. New York: Academic Press, 1975.

Hutchinson, Ann. *Labanotation*. New York: Dance Notation Bureau, 1970.

Kandinsky, Wassily. *Concerning the Spiritual in Art*. New York: Wittenborn, Schultz, Inc. 1947.

Kaplan, H. Roy. The M.L. Seidman Memorial Town Hall Lecture at Rhodes College. Memphis: March 1981.

Jianou, Ionel and Goldscheider, C. *Rodin*. Paris: Arted, 1969.

Leiris, Michel and Delange, Jacqueline. *African Art*. London: Thames and Hudson, 1968.

Marks, L.E. *Sensory Processes: The New Psychophysics*. New York: Academic Press. 1974.

McCarter, William and Gilbert, Rita. *Living with Art*. New York: Alfred A. Knopf, 1985.

Morris, William. *Hopes and Fears in Art: Collected Works of William Morris.* London: Longmans, Green and Co., 1914.

Munro, Thomas. *The Arts and Their Interrelationships.* Cleveland: The Press of Case Western Reserve University, 1967.

Ornstein, Robert and Sobel, David. *Healthy Pleasures.* Reading, Mass: Addison-Wesley, 1989.

Pepper, Stephen C. *Principles of Art Appreciation.* New York: Harcourt, Brace and World, Inc., 1949.

Picon, Gaeton. *Modern Painting: From 1800 to the Present.* New York: Newsweek Books, 1974.

Sage, George. *Introduction to Motor Behavior.* Reading, Mass: Addison-Wesley, 1977.

Shawn, Ted. *Every Little Movement.* Brooklyn: Dance Horizons, 1954.

Serra, Pere A. *Miró and Mallorca.* New York: Rizzoli, 1986.

Sheehan, George. *Running and Being.* New York: Simon and Schuster, 1978.

Wilson, David and Klindt-Jensen, Ole. *Viking Art.* London: George Allen and Unwin, 1966.

INDEX

CHRONIMED PUBLISHING
BOOKS OF RELATED INTEREST

Fat Is Not a Four-Letter Word by Charles Roy Schroeder, Ph.D. Through interesting scientific, nutritional, and historical evidence, this controversial and insightful guide shows why millions of "overweight" people are unnecessarily knocking themselves out to look like fashion models. It offers a realistic approach to healthful dieting and exercise.
004095 ISBN 1-56561-000-8 $14.95 ☐

Convenience Food Facts by Arlene Monk, R.D., C.D.E., with an introduction by Marion Franz, R.D., M.S. Includes complete nutrition information, tips, and exchange values on more than 1,500 popular name brand processed foods commonly found in grocery store freezers and shelves. Helps you plan easy-to-prepare, nutritious meals.
004081 ISBN 0-937721-77-8 $10.95 ☐

Fast Food Facts, Revised and Expanded Edition by Marion Franz, R.D., M.S. This revised and up-to-date best-seller shows how to make smart nutrition choices at fast food restaurants—and tells what to avoid. Includes complete nutrition information on more than 1,500 menu offerings from the 37 largest fast food chains.
Standard-size edition 004240 ISBN 1-56561-043-1 $7.95 ☐
Pocket edition 004229 ISBN 1-56561-031-8 $4.95 ☐

The Healthy Eater's Guide to Family & Chain Restaurants by Hope S. Warshaw, M.M.Sc., R.D. Here's the only guide that tells you how to eat healthier in over 100 of America's most popular family and chain restaurants. It offers complete and up-to-date nutrition information and suggests which items to choose and avoid.
004214 ISBN 1-56561-017-2 $9.95 ☐

Exchanges for All Occasions by Marion Franz, R.D., M.S. Exchanges and meal planning suggestions for just about any occasion, sample meal plans, special tips for people with diabetes, and more.
004201 ISBN 1-56561-005-9 $12.95 ☐

366 Low-Fat Brand-Name Recipes in Minutes by M. J. Smith, M.A., R.D./L.D. Here's more than a year's worth of the fastest family favorites using the country's most popular brand-name foods—from Minute Rice® to Ore Ida®—while reducing unwanted calories, fat, salt and cholesterol.
004247 ISBN 1-56561-050-4 $9.95 ☐

Fight Fat & Win, Updated & Revised Edition by Elaine Moquette-Magee, R.D., M.P.H. This breakthrough book explains how to easily incorporate low-fat dietary guidelines into every modern eating experience, from fast food and common restaurants to quick meals at home, simply by making smarter choices.
004244 ISBN 1-56561-047-4 $9.95 ☐

All-American Low-Fat Meals in Minutes by M.J. Smith R.D., L.D., M.A. Filled with tantalizing recipes and valuable tips, this cookbook makes great-tasting low-fat foods a snap for holidays, special occasions, or everyday. Most recipes take only minutes to prepare.

004079 ISBN 0-937721-73-5 $12.95 ☐

One Year of Healthy, Hearty, and Simple One-Dish Meals by Pam Spaude and Jan Owan-McMenamin, R.D., is a collection of 365 easy-to-make healthy and tasty family favorites and unique creations that are meals in themselves. Most of the dishes take under 30 minutes to prepare.

004217 ISBN 1-56561-019-9 $12.95 ☐

200 Kid-Tested Ways to Lower the Fat in Your Child's Favorite Foods by Elaine Moquette-Magee, M.P.H., R.D. For the first time ever, here's a much needed and asked for guide that gives easy, step-by-step instructions on cutting the fat in the most popular brand name and homemade foods kids eat every day–without them even noticing.

004231 ISBN 1-56561-034-2 $12.95 ☐

60 Days of Low-Fat, Low-Cost Meals in Minutes by M.J. Smith, R.D., L.D., M.A. Following the path of the best-seller *All American Low-Fat Meals in Minutes,* here are more than 150 quick and sumptuous recipes complete with the latest exchange values and nutrition facts for lowering calories, fat, salt, and cholesterol. This book contains complete menus for 60 days and recipes that use only ingredients found in virtually any grocery store—most for a total cost of less than $10.

004205 ISBN 1-56561-010-5 $12.95 ☐

CHRONIMED Publishing
P.O. Box 47945
Minneapolis, MN 55447-9727

Place a check mark next to the book (s) you would like sent. Enclosed is $____________. (Please add $3.00 to this order to cover postage and handling. Minnesota residents add 6.5% sales tax.) Send check or money order, no cash or C.O.D.'s. Prices are subject to change without notice.

Name ________________________________

Address ________________________________

City __________________ State _____ Zip ________

Allow 4 to 6 weeks for delivery.
Quantity discounts available upon request.
Or order by phone: 1-800-848-2793,
612-546-1146 (Minneapolis/St. Paul metro area).
Please have your credit card number ready.